Your First Year With Diabetes

THERESA GARNERO, APRN, BC-ADM, MSN, CDE

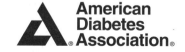

American Diabetes Association

Director, Book Publishing, Abe Ogden; *Managing Editor, Book Publishing,* Greg Guthrie; *Copyediting:* Cenveo Publisher Services; *Production Manager,* Melissa Sprott; *Composition,* ADA; *Illustrations,* Theresa Garnero; *Cover Design,* DropCap Design; *Printer,* Versa Press.

Printed in the United States of America
1 3 5 7 9 10 8 6 4 2

⊛ The paper in this publication meets the requirements of the ANSI Standard Z39.48-1992 (permanence of paper).

ADA titles may be purchased for business or promotional use or for special sales. To purchase more than 50 copies of this book at a discount, or for custom editions of this book with your logo, contact the American Diabetes Association at the address below, at booksales@diabetes.org, or by calling 703-299-2046.

American Diabetes Association
1701 North Beauregard Street
Alexandria, Virginia 22311

DOI: 10.2337/9781580404969

Library of Congress Cataloging-in-Publication Data

Garnero, Theresa.
   Your first year with diabetes : what to do, month by month / written and illustrated by Theresa Garnero, APRN, BC-ADM, MSN, CDE. -- Second edition.
      pages cm
   Includes bibliographical references and index.
   ISBN 978-1-58040-496-9 (alk. paper)
   1. Diabetes--Popular works. I. Title.
   RC660.4.G366 2013
   616.4'62--dc23
                          2012051158

Dedicated to people with diabetes and their caring community.

*Special thanks to all who have taught me about diabetes
and to the American Diabetes Association
for supporting this interactive book.*

CONTENTS

Month 4

Week 14	170
Week 15	174
Week 16	181
Week 17	185

Month 5

Week 18	190
Week 19	196
Week 20	201
Week 21	208

Month 6

Week 22	216
Week 23	225
Week 24	227
Week 25	230
Week 26	233

Month 7

Week 27	238
Week 28	244
Week 29	247
Week 30	249

Month 8

Week 31	252
Week 32	254
Week 33	259
Week 34	262

Introduction

Diabetes is about change—changing your life from the way it was and bringing changes to your whole being—mind, body, and spirit. You *can* be healthy with diabetes, especially if you are consistent. Every day presents ample opportunities to make decisions that affect your well-being. This interactive book is designed to help you learn the latest diabetes science so you can decide what to incorporate into your routine. As Dr. Elliot P. Joslin famously said, "The diabetic who knows the most, lives the longest." Yet, knowing and doing are two distinct entities. You can understand a topic, but for the science to have the best synergistic impact, you will need to pull apart the information and put back the pieces that are useful for your specific situation.

The more you adjust and cope with having diabetes, the better you will be able to take things in stride and care for yourself. And despite your best efforts, diabetes management is demanding and rarely predictable, neat, or tidy. It requires paying attention to detail, while trying to maintain a positive attitude—and sometimes you just don't feel like it. It's easy to get overwhelmed. You will have successes and you will have slip-ups—that's normal. It's a process that takes time and practice, and you don't have to be perfect! Just be patient with yourself, be your own champion, and lean on your circle of support when needed. Although this book is geared toward people with type 2 diabetes, many of the self-care management tips will apply to all types of diabetes. You also will find some product-related information, comparisons of brand names of food, and websites that may be helpful. Please know that I do not receive any financial incentives to provide this information and the American Diabetes Association does not endorse any of these products or supplies; I personally have checked out the resources so you can have a greater level of comfort when making up your own mind. Please ask your health-care provider for specific recommendations.

It is my honor to be involved even remotely with your journey and to share my unique perspective as a certified diabetes educator and humorist who knows the latest research and, equally as important, has experience with the real-life situations shared with me by thousands of people and their families dealing with diabetes. This repository of blended information offers you a positive approach to managing your diabetes and includes light-hearted humor. The art is in how you apply it to your everyday life while you continue to thrive in all the passions that keep you going.

Let's get started!

How to Use This Book

Have you noticed the icons? These health symbols represent the self-care behaviors that will help you navigate this book and your diabetes. You can easily identify a self-care behavior based on the symbols. At the end of each section, choose what to focus on or write in your own goal, and reflect on your progress. Health benefits happen by making small changes over time. And it's never too late to begin.

Symbol	Related key to diabetes self-management
	Eat wisely
	Be active
	Check numbers (includes glucose/A1C, blood pressure, cholesterol, and weight)
	Reduce stress
	Understand medications
	Solve problems
	Reduce risks
	Add humor

Source: Adapted from the AADE 7™ Self-Care Behaviors.

Your First Year with Diabetes Roadmap

Another way to look at the year ahead and understand how the book works is to consider this schematic. Topics are presented in a need-to-know order that will have the biggest impact, will address safety, and will build in steps for success. You will reflect on goals and achievements with interactive activities and quarterly reviews. As the weeks and months continue, you will be presented with deeper layers of science and shared knowledge.

When multiple topics are offered in a given week or month, review each one to see if it is relevant and important to you. If it is, you read the details, decide whether you'd like to take action by incorporating or continuing current behaviors, and whether you need help staying motivated. If not, you move to the next topic. Diabetes care is vast and everyone has a unique situation, so some topics will have more relevance than others. This book is flexible in its setup. Use the index to skip ahead to a topic that is urgent for your situation.

Along the way, you will learn about standards of care and tips to refine your abilities as well as ongoing resources that will be helpful for your first year and beyond.

Your First Year with Diabetes Roadmap

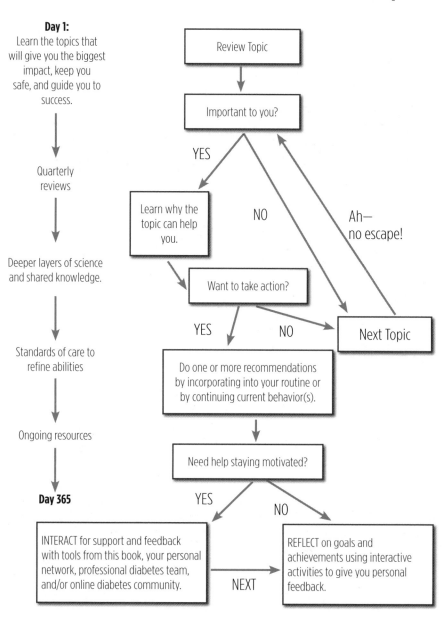

Day 1:
Learn the topics that will give you the biggest impact, keep you safe, and guide you to success.

Quarterly reviews

Deeper layers of science and shared knowledge.

Standards of care to refine abilities

Ongoing resources

Day 365

Review Topic

Important to you?

YES

NO

Ah—
no escape!

Learn why the topic can help you.

Want to take action?

YES

NO

Next Topic

Do one or more recommendations by incorporating into your routine or by continuing current behavior(s).

Need help staying motivated?

YES

NO

INTERACT for support and feedback with tools from this book, your personal network, professional diabetes team, and/or online diabetes community.

NEXT

REFLECT on goals and achievements using interactive activities to give you personal feedback.

WEEK 1

Laughin' Langerhans   *By Theresa Garnero*

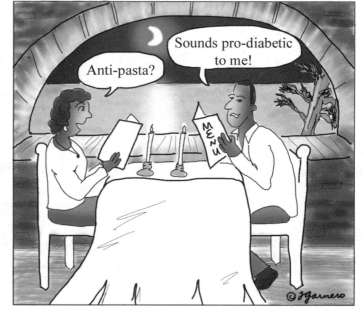

DAY 1

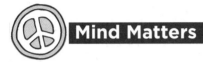

Mind Matters

I was told I might have diabetes—now what?

Take a deep breath. Preparing your mind for your journey with diabetes is one of the best first steps to take. Being told you have diabetes, or that there is a problem with your blood glucose level, or that you have prediabetes can cause quite a bit of stress—and rightly so.

Diabetes can be scary. You may have read headlines about what can go wrong or witnessed firsthand the negative effects of uncontrolled diabetes. Maybe you have been in denial that anything is wrong. That's okay. Denial protects and buffers you from difficult or shocking information. Do you feel guilty? Like you caused diabetes? If so, your first assignment is to stop the blame game and get on your own side. Anger, too, is a common reaction and is often the first sign that you acknowledge that something is wrong. It is never too late to jump start your diabetes self-management program. The key is to be gentle with yourself because you are your best resource for managing your diabetes.

Diabetes is never convenient, but with some effort, help from the experts, and support from your personal community, it is manageable. It is important that you acknowledge this. How you perceive this diagnosis will greatly affect the level of success with which your diabetes is managed. Your thoughts and feelings have an enormous impact on the body. Positive thoughts have positive physiologic repercussions in the body. So let's check in with your current emotional state. Why? Making and maintaining a change often depends on your emotional state. Which one of the statements opposite rings true for you now?

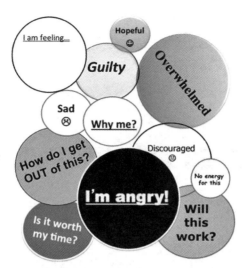

Your feelings about diabetes will change day by day. All emotions are fair game. What you do with them is up to you. What are some ways you are willing to deal with the stress of your diabetes diagnosis today?

PERSONAL GOAL

Jot down today's date: _____ I will:

☐ Allow myself to be angry over my loss of spontaneity.
☐ Take a time out: see a movie; go for a walk or scenic drive; meditate.
☐ Listen to a favorite piece of music.
☐ Start a journal.
☐ Stop harping on myself.
☐ Plan on imperfection (in both daily life and life with diabetes).
☐ Close my eyes, take a deep breath, and go on a 2-minute vacation, visualizing my favorite getaway spot.
☐ Enjoy a bubble bath.
☐ Find five things that bring me joy.
☐ Other: _____.

 The good news is that I am coping. The bad news is that I maxed out my credit card!

DAY
2

Diagnosis: Diabetes

What is diabetes?

Although diabetes means you have too much blood glucose, it is the end result of a complex, hormonal issue that relates to the body's ability to make and use insulin and to get energy from foods.

When we eat, food eventually turns into glucose, the main source of energy for the millions of microscopic cells in our body. The only way for the cells to get this glucose is with insulin. Insulin is made by specialized beta-cells within the pancreas. The pancreas is a gland situated behind the stomach. It releases insulin into the bloodstream in response to the blood glucose rise after meals and snacks. Insulin is the key that unlocks the cell door to allow the glucose to enter where it is used for energy.

In people with diabetes, the pancreas is on an early retirement plan, so less insulin is available in the body. In addition, the body doesn't use the remaining insulin well, resulting in glucose piling up in the bloodstream. If left uncontrolled, these high levels of glucose in the blood eventually cause problems throughout the body. Luckily, you can change the course of this disease and prevent the laundry list of possible complications through your everyday behaviors. You can even be the healthiest person on your block.

Understandably, you may be worried about the risk of getting diabetes-related complications. Diabetes health comes from applying relevant research and professional knowledge to your individual experience and everyday efforts. Some of the risk for complications is controlled by genetic factors, so you do your best on a daily basis to combine what is in your control (your "environment"—sensible eating, being active, and, if needed, taking medications) with what is not under your control (your "genetics" or inherited traits from your parents and ancestors).

By the time type 2 diabetes is diagnosed, up to 80% of the beta-cells may be destroyed. You can help protect your remaining beta-cells by making mindful food choices, being active on a regular basis, and, when needed, taking medication. Compounding the issue is insulin resistance, which is common with type 2 diabetes and often occurs with individuals who are overweight. When someone has insulin resistance, cells do not respond to circulating insulin (whether the insulin was released from the pancreas or taken in the form of an injection). This means "the lock" on the cell is stubborn and insulin ("the key") has difficulty opening it, thus blood glucose levels go up. Left untreated, blood glucose levels go even higher. Lack of exercise, obesity, smoking and secondhand smoke, high blood glucose, sleep problems, stress, and hereditary factors all play a role in the development of insulin resistance.

> **Some Language Trivia**
>
> Our word "diabetes" originally comes from the Greek word for "siphon." When blood glucose levels are high, water is pulled from the cells and put into the bloodstream, which explains why some people have increased thirst and urination as symptoms.

The gray zone: prediabetes

Prediabetes is a condition in which glucose levels are rising but are not high enough to be categorized as type 2 diabetes. (See the section "How is it diagnosed?") Research has shown that people with prediabetes are at a high risk for developing type 2 diabetes, which often can be prevented or delayed by getting 150 minutes of physical activity a week (e.g., 30 minutes of physical activity 5 days a week) and for those who are overweight, by losing 7% of weight (e.g., if you weighed 200 pounds, that would mean losing 14 pounds to reduce your weight by 7%).

Why did I get diabetes?

No one can be sure. Even though millions of people have it, each individual's case is different. Some scientific theories suggest that an environmental trigger activates a genetic code, flipping the diabetes switch to "on."

How did I get diabetes? I don't eat a lot of sugar.

It is not as simple as sugar consumption. It's part genetics and environment, and sometimes the cause is not known.

In terms of genetics, do you have any immediate relatives with diabetes? Recent studies have shown that many people have diabetes for 7 years before they are diagnosed, so family history of the disease is not always obvious. Have any of your relatives suffered a heart attack or a stroke? Either could arise from undiagnosed type 2 diabetes. Many people with type 2 diabetes do not have any signs or symptoms of the disease before getting diagnosed.

In terms of environment, did you know drinking just one soda per day may increase the risk of diabetes? If you gain weight from consuming too many calories (whether from sugar or something else) or lack of physical activity, and if you have a genetic predisposition for diabetes, then that can trigger it.

What type of diabetes do I have?

There are many types of diabetes, including type 1 diabetes, type 2 diabetes, latent autoimmune diabetes in adults (LADA), and gestational diabetes (also known as hyperglycemia during pregnancy).

How is it diagnosed?

Diabetes is diagnosed by measuring laboratory blood glucose levels in one of the three following ways*:
1. Fasting glucose: blood taken first thing in the morning after no food or calorie-containing drinks for at least 8 hours.
2. Nonfasting glucose: blood taken at any time of the day, regardless of what you ate or drank.
3. A1C or estimated glucose average: an average blood glucose from the last 3 months.

For diagnosis	Fasting glucose	Nonfasting glucose†	A1C
No diabetes	99 mg/dL or less	139 mg/dL or less	5.6% or less
Prediabetes	100–125 mg/dL	140–199 mg/dL	5.7–6.4%
Diabetes	126 mg/dL or more	200 mg/dL or more	6.5% or more

†Nonfasting glucose is a 2-hour blood glucose value taken after 75 grams of glucose consumed during an oral glucose tolerance test (OGTT).

*If the initial test does not show clear levels of high blood glucose, results should be confirmed by repeat testing.

Knowing which type of diabetes you have helps you get the proper treatment. After talking to my health-care provider, I discovered that I have this type of diabetes: _____

Is diabetes contagious?

No, diabetes is not contagious. You cannot catch diabetes from someone or give it to someone you know. Your relatives may have "given" it to you through your genes, but that is very different from catching a cold.

The almighty A1C

The gold standard for checking overall diabetes management is a blood test called the A1C test (often referred to as HbA_{1c} or hemoglobin A1C). It measures your average blood glucose levels over a 3-month period and is reported as a percentage (%), or an estimated average glucose (eAG). On your lab printout, you may find the eAG, which expresses A1C in the same units as glucose meters (mg/dL). This is intended to make it easier to understand how the A1C relates to your glucose values.

The A1C test measures how much glucose is stuck to the hemoglobin part of the red blood cell. Red blood cells live for 2–3 months, carry oxygen and nutrients throughout the bloodstream, and carry away the waste. When a glucose molecule is nearby, it attaches to the red blood cell and won't let go; that's how we can tell what has happened for the past 3 months. The goal for many people newly diagnosed with diabetes is to have an A1C of less than 7%. An A1C of 7% compares to an average blood glucose level of 154 mg/dL. Talk with your provider about your individualized A1C goal. Less stringent A1C goals may be appropriate for those with a history of severe low blood glucose (discussed on day 10), the very young, limited life expectancy, those with long-standing diabetes difficult to control, or those with other conditions (such as cardiovascular disease or complications, such as eye and kidney-related disease). Also, consider that if a person is anemic, for example, he or she will have fewer red blood cells, rendering an A1C test inaccurate.

It is typical to have a high A1C when you are first diagnosed and to have the value fluctuate over the years. Keep in mind that even

Type 2 Diabetes

Type 2 diabetes is the most common type of diabetes and is caused by the body's resistance to insulin and a decline of insulin production. Type 2 diabetes typically arises in adults (occurring most often in 45- to 64-year-olds); children and teenagers also may develop type 2 diabetes, especially if they are overweight and have a family history of diabetes. Treatment often requires medication (including pills, injectable medication, or insulin). The symptoms often are subtle, varying from none to tiredness (especially after a large meal), blurred vision, frequent urination at night, and dry, itchy skin.

Type 1 Diabetes

Type 1 diabetes is an autoimmune disorder in which the body mistakenly destroys the insulin-producing beta-cells, causing insulin deficiency. Type 1 diabetes was once called juvenile diabetes because most diagnoses occur with children and young adults, but not always. Insulin therapy is required. Additional laboratory tests used to check for type 1 diabetes include C-peptide, islet cell antibodies (ICA), insulin auto-antibodies (IAA), glutamic acid decarboxylase (GAD), and zinc transporter 8 (ZnT8). The symptoms of type 1 diabetes are typically obvious: profound thirst, frequent urination, hunger, and rapid weight loss, and may include nausea, vomiting, or abdominal pain, a hard time breathing, fruity odor on breath, and confusion.

Latent Autoimmune Diabetes in Adults

Latent autoimmune diabetes in adults (LADA) has components of both type 1 and type 2 diabetes. The auto-antibodies that cause beta-cell failure are present, but the process is slow. Individuals with LADA often are misdiagnosed with type 2 diabetes and only go on insulin therapy after oral medications are proven ineffective. If you were mistakenly diagnosed with type 2 diabetes under the age of 50 years, have a BMI of less than 25 kg/m2, are not responding to diabetes pills, or have a personal or family history of autoimmune disease, ask to have your islet cell antibodies checked.

Gestational Diabetes

Gestational diabetes is a condition in which high glucose levels start or are recognized during pregnancy. Pregnant women typically are screened for this at 24–28 weeks gestation. Treatment includes carbohydrate counting, glucose self-monitoring, exercise, and medication or insulin. Maintaining optimal glucose levels prevents problems (baby growing more than 9 pounds, risk for delivery complications, or, later, childhood obesity and type 2 diabetes). Because there is a rapid increase in the cumulative incidence of type 2 diabetes occurring in the first 5 years after delivery, maintaining a healthy body weight (by losing weight if needed or preventing weight gain) through mindful eating and being active, helps to prevent or delay type 2 diabetes.

though the A1C is a very important number, it does not define you or all of your efforts to be healthy with diabetes.

PERSONAL GOAL

Date: _____ I will:

☐ Ask my doctor's office for copies of my laboratory tests (blood glucose and A1C) to learn what results got me the diagnosis.

☐ Get organized with my health records by keeping all lab results and important contact information in a binder (or file them electronically in such a way you can actually find them later).

☐ Ask to have an A1C blood test (if not done in the past 3 months).

☐ Acknowledge that I have diabetes.

☐ Reach out to someone I trust for encouragement.

☐ Calm my mind with three deep breaths.

☐ Other: _____.

It's official. I'm really sweet!

DAY
3

Eat Wisely

What can I eat?

Living successfully with diabetes is about making wise food choices more times than not without compromising the joy surrounding mealtime. But it's easier said than done. We are creatures of habit. We are used to doing things a certain way. It's not about eating like a saint—it's about making small changes over time to eat more nutritiously. It's a process, not an event.

The step-by-step guide that follows gives you small bites of information at a time. We'll start with general concepts and specific take-home points that you can start using today, with more and more details unfolding throughout the months ahead. What actions are you willing to consider from the diabetes education buffet? Below are suggestions backed by research that you can incorporate into your daily life.

Eat Better and Feel the Difference!

After you eat, your blood glucose level goes up. Foods containing carbohydrates (also known as "carbs") raise glucose the most. A lot of people are fearful of carbs as a result. We need carbohydrates for brain function and energy, so please don't cut them out entirely!

1. You *can* have carbohydrates, but stick with sensible portion sizes that are consistent from day to day.
2. Choose a variety of foods that are rich in vitamins and minerals and low in calories.
3. Eat regularly; this means three meals a day and snacks, if needed, 2–3 hours after a meal.
4. Skipping meals may cause blood glucose fluctuations and eating too much late in the day may cause weight gain.

5. Products that claim that they have "No Added Sugar" or are "Sugar Free" often still have carbs!
6. Check food labels (i.e., the Nutrition Facts label) for serving size and the total carbohydrate amount to start learning about carbs.
7. See a registered dietitian who has an expertise in diabetes (often this is a certified diabetes educator) for an individual meal plan.

	Choose often	Choose less often
Preparation methods	Bake, broil, roast, steam, grill	Fried
Breads/grains*	Whole grains, specifically: brown rice, barley, whole-wheat bread, oatmeal, wild rice, small whole-grain bagels, and bulgur	White bread, muffins, croissants, biscuits, white rice, French bread, and sweetened cereals
Starchy vegetables*	Peas, corn, winter squash, baked/mashed/boiled potato	French fries, instant mashed potatoes
Nonstarchy vegetables	Broccoli, bell peppers, mushrooms, zucchini, celery, spinach, eggplant, and greens	Tempura or fried vegetables with added fat, vegetables in sauces
Fruits*	Whole fruits (small portions), dried fruits without added sugar, and frozen fruit	Juice: regular or with added sugar (eat fruit instead, or add water to dilute it); canned fruit with added sugar (if this is more affordable for you, be sure to rinse it first)
Milk/dairy*	Nonfat plain or Greek yogurt, no-sugar-added light yogurt, nonfat or low-fat milk	Whole milk, half and half, ice cream, milk shakes, low-fat sweetened or regular yogurt
Meat and meat alternatives	Skinless, white poultry, lean beef/pork (trim off fat); fish/seafood; natural peanut butter, tofu/gluten†, legumes* (beans, peas, lentils)	Bacon, sausage, ham, luncheon meats, poultry skins, fatty meats, hard cheeses, breaded* or fried fish/chicken/meats/tofu/gluten

	Choose often	Choose less often
Fats, oils, seasonings	Liquid oils (canola, olive), soft tub margarines without trans fat, nuts in small amounts, 1/8 avocado	Butter, lard, solid fats, sour cream, mayonnaise, tropical oils (palm, palm kernel, coconut)
Sweeteners, condiments*	Only as desired sugar substitutes: Stevia, Zero (xylitol), Splenda (sucralose), NutraSweet or Equal (aspartame), Sweet 'N Low (saccharin); sugar-free syrups/jams/jellies†	Avoid added fructose (but not fruit) and fructose corn syrup‡ Limit table sugar, honey, syrup, regular jams/jellies* as they have no nutritional value and have carbs
Desserts*, Beverages†	Water is best, diet sodas or other sugar-free beverages in order to wean off regular sodas; not to choose often but to use in place of regular desserts or candy: fruit-based desserts, sugar-free candies, diet pudding, sugar-free Jell-O	Regular soda, juice, hot chocolate, donuts, pastries, cake, pie, candy, sherbet, ice cream, cookies

*Contains carbohydrates; †may contain carbohydrates; ‡recent controversial research suggests that fructose converts to fat more easily and increases insulin resistance, although a consensus has still not been reached by the scientific community.

Free Foods

Foods containing less than 20 calories per serving and fewer than 5 grams of carbohydrate count as a "free food" (unless you eat more than the recommended serving, in which case, they are not free). Here is a short list of free foods.

- 1/4 cup of salsa
- 1 tablespoon of salad dressing or catsup
- sugar-free gelatin or gum
- sugar substitutes
- salad greens
- diet soft drinks
- vinegar
- lemon juice
- seasonings
- nonfat cooking spray
- tea and coffee
- 1/2 cup of blueberries
- water

PERSONAL GOAL

Date: _____ I will:

☐ Make time for breakfast every day (even if it's something small).
   What I had for breakfast was: _____

_____

☐ Eat three small meals a day and a little snack if I get hungry.
☐ Try not to skip meals.
☐ Ask myself while eating, "Am I satisfied or stuffed?"
☐ Focus on savoring flavors.
☐ Add a serving of veggies to my main meal.
☐ Cut my consumption in half of (pick one or more): regular soda, juice, alcohol, candy, cookies, ice cream, pastries, cakes, or anything deep fried.
☐ Select 100% whole-wheat instead of white bread.
☐ Choose fresh fruit for dessert.
☐ Replace regular sugar with a sugar substitute.
☐ Other: _____.

I eat often.
With Barbie-doll dishes,
I have no choice!

DAY
4

Get Active

Who has the time to exercise? I am simply too busy.

Making time for health is challenging. You are in charge of your over-all well-being. As the project manager of your health, are you making an *informed* decision when you opt out of physical activity? Exercise is the single most underutilized self-care behavior that can make a dif-ference in all things diabetes and health in general.

What kinds of activities will help my diabetes?

The world is your oyster! The basic principle is to pick a physical activity that you enjoy that is fun, nearby, and easy to do. The gym is great for some people; others prefer getting outdoors! Invite a friend or the entire family. If you haven't been exercising, start slowly and avoid extreme activity levels. Be sure to warm up and cool down. Going from zero exercise to an hour at the gym every day, when you haven't been to it in years, can lead to injury and dis-courage you from sticking with your activity plan.

Being active

- Improves blood glucose levels and insulin sensitivity
- Helps you lose weight or maintain weight loss
- Lowers blood pressure and stress
- Raises good cholesterol levels (high-density lipoprotein [HDL])
- Improves heart function, sex life, and sleep
- Helps to prevent and manage depression
- Keeps bones healthy
- Increases life span
- Saves money (fewer health issues and less medicine mean more money in your pocket)

Do I really need a cardiac stress test?

Recent guidelines from the American Diabetes Association conclude that routine screening is not recommended. Your health-care provider will use clinical judgment based on the following risk factors*:

- Sedentary and 35 years or older
- Sedentary with diabetes for more than 10 years
- Had type 2 diabetes for more than 10 years or type 1 diabetes for more than 15 years
- Have a family history of premature coronary artery disease (a heart-related event in a first-degree relative that happens at less than 60 years of age)
- Heart or blood vessel disease
- High blood pressure
- High cholesterol
- Smoking/exposure to secondhand smoke
- Obesity
- Peripheral vascular disease (PVD)
- Chest pain or discomfort during exercise
- Severe eye disease (called proliferative diabetic retinopathy)
- Severe nerve system disease (autonomic neuropathy, or peripheral neuropathy, or history of foot lesions)

Source: American Diabetes Association Clinical Practice Guidelines, 2013, and "Exercise Manual: An Exercise Guide for Adults with Diabetes," 2nd ed. by Richard Peng, MS, MBA, ACSM-RCEP, CDE.

PERSONAL GOAL

Date: _____ I will:

☐ Take the stairs instead of the elevator.
☐ Get off at an earlier bus stop and walk a little farther.
☐ Park the car farther away.
☐ Stretch my muscles for 5 minutes in the morning.
☐ Walk the dog around the block.
☐ Do leg squats while curling my hair.
☐ Lift a small soup can 10 times in each hand while watching television.
☐ Talk with my provider about whether it would be appropriate for me to have a cardiac stress test.
☐ Other: _____.

 Walking—it's not just for the dogs!

DAY 5

 Check Glucose

My doctor said I need to poke my finger. Is it really necessary?

Self-monitoring of blood glucose (SMBG) is the best way to get immediate feedback on your food choices and to know whether you are protected against the consequences of uncontrolled diabetes. Would you withdraw money without knowing the balance of your account? Well, maybe if you're rich, but this is your health. So for many people, it is very helpful.

What does blood glucose testing involve?

You'll need a clean pair of hands and a home blood glucose monitoring kit, including the following:

- Blood glucose monitor—a small device that analyzes your blood glucose value within seconds.
- Lancet device—another name for a needle holder, which helps you poke your finger or arm. Once you two become acquainted, you can call it the "poker."
- Lancet—a name for a small needle.
- Test strip—a thin piece of plastic on which you place a tiny drop of blood that is next placed inside the monitor.

Are you a little freaked out by the notion of needles? That's normal. Luckily, the diabetes industry has vastly improved the lancing devices and everything else related to SMBG. This allows you to get a drop of blood with little to no pain.

Purchase lancets with small needle widths (gauges size 30 and up are narrower). Turn the lancet device down to the necessary depth to get blood. Prick the side of your finger where there are fewer nerve endings and, therefore, less pain. Rotate fingertips. If you use the same two or three victims each time, you'll develop calluses that will make it harder to get enough blood. Also, hang your hand below your heart and squeeze the base of the finger, sending more blood toward your fingertip. This makes getting a proper blood sample easier.

How do I get the right meter for me and learn how to use it?

With so many different meters on the market, you need help to find the one that's right for you. Do you need something simple or sophisticated? How do you work the thing? Which one is covered by your health plan?

Each health insurance plan has preferred meters that are covered with a prescription. You can make a cup of tea, sit down, and contact your insurance company to find out which glucose meter they prefer. Without a prescription, the test strips are expensive, so start with a meter covered by your insurance company (Medicare allows nearly all systems). Several companies provide mail-order supply delivery and bill your insurance directly. If you do not have insurance, ask your health-care provider or certified diabetes educator (CDE) for a free meter or if they know of any other local resources.

A CDE can help you make the best meter choice and guide you in making a strategy for your ongoing health. CDEs specialize in diabetes self-management. According to the American Diabetes Association, at the time of diagnosis, people with diabetes should receive diabetes self-management education. You can find a CDE in your area by calling 800-832-6874 or by checking the American Association of Diabetes Educators website at www.diabeteseducator.org and clicking on "Find an Educator." Or find an American Diabetes Association Recognized Education Program by visiting http://professional.diabetes.org/erp_list.aspx.

When do I test?

You have many chances. You can check before and 2 hours after meals, before and after exercise, before you drive, before you take an exam, before bedtime, when medicines change, when you feel low, or when you don't feel well. Your health-care provider can work out an individualized plan. Start simple, with tests two times a day.

> **Option 1:** Test fasting (immediately after waking in the morning) and 2 hours after breakfast.
> **Option 2:** Test before dinner and 2 hours after dinner.

Record your results for a few weeks and look for patterns of glucose readings at a particular time. Are the numbers all over the place? Ask your diabetes educator for help interpreting the patterns; otherwise, checking glucose can be *enormously* frustrating. Plus, studies have shown that the more data you share with your providers, the better care you'll get and your diabetes control will improve in turn. One study found that people with type 2 diabetes who tested their blood glucose more than once daily and people with type 1 diabetes who tested more than three times daily had an A1C that was on average 1% lower than those who did not.

The inside scoop

If your blood glucose level goes up less than 50 mg/dL from before the meal to 2 hours after, your body can manage the carbohydrates in that meal. For example, let's say your before-breakfast reading was 200 and your after-breakfast reading was 240. The baseline level of 200 is too high (which often happens with new diagnosis) but the meal was okay (in terms of your body's response to the carbohydrate content). In this example, if you did not know the baseline number of 200, you might assume the food you had for your breakfast was not good. If all of this is too much to digest, forge ahead. There is plenty of time to understand what your results mean.

Another tip: Losing 7% of your current weight (if you are overweight) can lower glucose levels, as does a daily 20-minute walk. Chip away at this by eating 100 calories less every day. In a year, that adds up to 10 pounds! These things do not happen overnight, unless you are a movie star with a great plastic surgeon.

What is the target range?

Blood glucose level ideal ranges* are as follows:

Before a meal (called preprandial): 70–130 mg/dL
2 hours after a meal (called postprandial): less than 180 mg/dL

---

*Your health-care team may create a slightly different range to meet your specific needs.

Where can I throw away lancets?

Many states have specific laws making it illegal to throw sharps waste in the trash, and require an approved sharps container. You wouldn't want someone to get injured from a lancet tossed in the trash! Ask your waste disposal company about local laws and if a needle disposal program is available. Some pharmacies accept full sharps containers with free replacements.

PERSONAL GOAL

Date: _____ I will:

☐ Obtain a blood glucose meter within 1 week.

☐ Open up that blood glucose meter kit and start learning how to check my levels or call the toll-free assistance line on the back of the meter.

☐ Ask for a referral to see a local CDE.

☐ Check my glucose before breakfast and 2 hours after breakfast, and record the results for 1 week.

☐ Test my blood glucose before dinner and 2 hours after dinner, and record the results for 1 week.

☐ Other: _____.

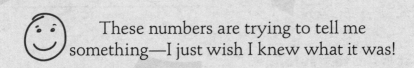

These numbers are trying to tell me something—I just wish I knew what it was!

DAY 6

A Tough Pill to Swallow

I don't want to start taking pills. Once you start, you never stop, right?

It's not necessarily true that you'll be taking pills forever. They help get your glucose levels close to or within the target ranges as quickly as possible and that helps you prevent complications.

Diabetes is a progressive disease (which means that it can gradually worsen over time) and usually requires some medication at one point or another. If your health-care team recommends medication, it's not because you are failing with your diet or exercise; your pancreas is failing. We use beauty products to improve how we look on the outside. Why not help our body on the inside, too?

How can I motivate myself to take my medication as instructed?

Do you understand the risks and benefits? (Diabetes medication reviewed on Day 12.) Are you having trouble with the expense, side effects, or remembering to take them? Involve your health-care provider so you can find a solution.

PERSONAL GOAL

Date: _____ I will:

☐ Consider that diabetes medications may help me live a longer, healthier life.

☐ Call my health-care provider, CDE, or pharmacist about any medication-related questions or side effects I'm having.

☐ Develop a system to help me remember to take my medicine (e.g., get a pill reminder, carry extra doses in my purse or briefcase, keep an extra dose at work, write down when I took them).

☐ Put pills where I'll remember to take them.

☐ Tell a trusted health-care provider that I am having trouble paying for my medications or ask the pharmacist about patient-assistance programs for any of my medications.

☐ Miss fewer doses of my medication.

☐ Ask my health-care provider for samples of my medication.

☐ Other: _____.

 I wanted early retirement, but my pancreas went without me.

DAY
7

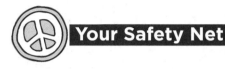 **Your Safety Net**

How am I supposed to manage this?

Diabetes can be tough sometimes, especially if you try to manage it always by yourself. Don't be afraid to ask for a little help from your friends, family, colleagues, and health-care team. Share the burden.

It can be a challenge finding people who are willing to be supportive to the degree that you need. You'll no doubt run into people in your immediate circle—perhaps even your partner—who don't want *anything* to do with your diabetes. To whom can you turn? Who will help you stay positive?

Decide whom to tell and whom to lean on for support. Tell them what you need. Do you want guidance about meal selections? Do you want them to go for walks with you? From a safety standpoint, you'll need to have someone who knows what to do in an emergency situation (such as what to do in case of low blood glucose, discussed in Week 2, Day 10). Moreover, it helps to have someone join you in your journey toward health. Who is willing to learn about carbohydrate counting with you? Who might join you in becoming more active? These are the people who may support you.

PERSONAL GOAL

Date: _____ I will:

☐ Talk with a trusted friend or family member about my diabetes.

☐ Seek out health-care professionals with whom I feel a bond.

☐ Discuss my diabetes with someone who has it to get a little more perspective. (Caution: Everyone has opinions about what a person with diabetes should or shouldn't do, some of which are medically incorrect. When getting medical advice, deal with health-care professionals.)

☐ Obtain a medical alert bracelet, necklace, or wallet card as part of my safety plan (a free one is available at www.diabeteswellness. net/WellnessNetwork/FREEDiabetesIDNecklace.aspx).

☐ Meditate or pray for 10 minutes.

☐ Look for support in groups to which I already belong.

☐ Avoid people who will not be supportive.

☐ Be grateful for all that I do have.

☐ Other: _____.

 Sure, they help me with my diabetes, but what about my garage sale?

WEEK 1: REVIEW

Date: _____

Look back at your personal goals. How successful were you at accomplishing what you set out to do?

☐ Mostly   ☐ Sometimes   ☐ Rarely
  (80% or more)   (50–80%)   (less than 50%)

Easiest

1. What was the easiest to achieve? _____

_____

2. Why? What helped make the difference? _____

_____

3. How can you ensure your continued success? _____

_____

Most challenging

1. What was the most challenging to achieve? _____

_____

2. Why? What barriers got in the way? _____

_____

3. What can you do to remove that barrier?_____

_____

WEEK 2

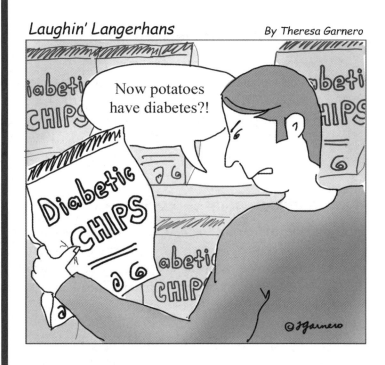

Laughin' Langerhans — By Theresa Garnero

DAY
8

Count, Don't Cut Out, Carbohydrates

What is a carbohydrate?

Commonly nicknamed "carbs," carbohydrates are an energy-rich nutrient found in fruits, grains, some vegetables, beans, milk, yogurt, and, of course, sweets, candy, and cookies. You may know these as "starches."

Why are carbohydrates important?

Carbs are the body's main source of energy and they raise blood glucose levels quickly, faster than fat or protein. Once a carb enters your mouth, it starts to convert into glucose, the fuel your entire body needs to function. Your brain needs glucose to function. That's why people who have glucose levels less than 70 mg/dL (called hypoglycemia) can act strangely; they are running out of fuel and brainpower.

How can I stop eating carbohydrates? I love them!

Don't cut them out! Instead, follow this carb-controlled approach to your diet. For people with diabetes, the issue is quality and quantity. We focus on carbs because they are the food group that raises glucose levels quicker than proteins and fats. It takes carbs only 15–90 minutes to convert into glucose in the bloodstream, whereas proteins can take hours.

The first step is to learn to identify a carbohydrate, which is the point of the next exercise. After that, you will begin learning about how carb portions affect blood glucose.

Check Your Carb Smarts!

Circle the foods below that contain carbohydrate.

Column 1	Column 2	Column 3	Column 4	Column 5
Small 1-ounce muffin	10–15 grapes	Egg	Avocado	Broccoli
1/3 cup of rice	Sliver of cake (1 ounce)	Chicken leg	Butter	Diet soda
1/3 cup pasta	4 ounces juice	Tofu	Oil	Mushrooms
1 slice whole-wheat bread	8 ounces of plain yogurt	Cheese	Chicken skin	Salad
1 cup of milk	Small ear of corn	Fish	Nuts	Water

Answer:

Columns 1 and 2: Foods and food portions with 15 grams of carbohydrate.
Column 3: Protein servings only, no carbohydrate.
Column 4: Fat servings, no carbohydrate.
Column 5: Free foods, no, or minimal, carbohydrate.

How many carbohydrates can I eat?

Everyone differs slightly in how much carbohydrate they can handle. An athlete needs and can burn many more carbohydrates than someone who gets less activity. A general guideline is to have the following:

- A total of 45–60 grams of carbohydrate per meal for men

- A total of 30–45 grams of carbohydrate per meal for women
- Approximately 15 grams of carb for snacks

The only way to know how many carbs are in a particular food is by looking at the food label (see the section "Nutrition Facts label") or in a carb reference guide (for foods that do not have labels, such as fresh fruit). Note that several smart phone apps have carb-counting databases, which are reviewed in Week 26. If counting carbs does not suit your fancy, check out the Plate Method on Day 15. It's a simple way to manage carb portions (no counting required!).

Can I save up my carbohydrates from one meal to the next?

Nice try, but no. Eating all of those carbs at one meal will have a profound impact on your glucose level. It would be too much for your pancreas to handle. Learning how to space out your carbs throughout the day will serve you well. It is the balance of carbohydrate consistency, taking medicine when needed, being active on most days, managing stress, and your remaining pancreas function that affect glucose control.

How can I keep track of all of this information?

Try using a log, such as the following one, to keep track of your eating habits, carbs, exercise, sleep patterns, and more. It is a proven way to lose weight! Start by tracking your food, then add other behaviors as you're ready to. (And yes, there's a smart phone app for that—reviewed in Week 26—but it is fine to start with the chart opposite.)

Food Detective

Here's a commonly voiced concern: "I'm afraid to eat because it might hurt my body." You won't hurt your body if you know what you're putting in it. With a little effort, learning about the food label (officially called the Nutrition Facts label) is one of the most powerful tools you'll use in putting together a healthy meal plan.

Just the (nutrition) facts, ma'am

Nutrition Facts labels are like price tags. Is the food you're thinking of buying rich in nutrients or are you getting ripped off? How can you tell?

1. **Start with the serving size.** Nearly everything that is writ-

Food and Activity Diary

You can keep track of your daily progress by noting the following:

Date:_____Weight:_____

Time	Food/Beverage	Amount	Calories	Carbs	Notes

Cross off each time I have an 8-ounce glass of water: 1 2 3 4 5

Hours of sleep last night:_____   Level of stress yesterday: low, medium, high

Type of physical activity: _____, Minutes:_____

How I did today: Fabulous____ Great____ Okay____ Will do better tomorrow____

ten on food packaging, including the Nutrition Facts label, is based on the serving size. Many people mistake the package as the portion size; this is referred to as "portion distortion." It's easy to double or triple calories, fat, and carbohydrate intake by eating the whole package at once. Also, the serving size listed on the label isn't necessarily the same serving size as you'll be using to count carbohydrates. For example, the label might say that the serving size of cooked rice is 1 cup, but 15 grams of carb is a 1/3 cup of rice.

2. **Check total carbohydrates.** Focus on the grams of total carbohydrate, not the percentage. Many people also fall into the trap of dwelling only on the sugars in a food. A product can be sugar free and still have lots of carbohydrate (e.g., sugar-free cookies made with flour).

3. **Calories and calories from fat.** Here's a way to distinguish between calories and calories from fat. They are like miles per gallon in the city versus the highway. If a food choice has only 100 calories, but 85 of those calories are from fat, your arteries and waistline may suffer if you frequently choose it. As a general rule, no more than 35%

How many calories do I need a day?

Your calorie needs depend on your age, sex, body size (height/weight), and activity level. To maintain your current weight, check out this online calorie chart that gives you specifics: www.diabetes.org/assets/pdfs/2010-calorie-intake-chart.pdf.

But let's take an example so you can get the idea of how this works. To *maintain* current weight, the caloric needs of a 51- to 55-year-old woman are 1,600 calories if she is sedentary, 1,800 if she's moderately active, and 2,200 if she's very active. The same-age man gets 2,200 if he's sedentary, 2,400 if he's moderately active, and 2,800 if he's very active. Women get shortchanged again! (We don't have the muscle mass that men do and therefore don't need as many calories.) This is a guide and a tool, but let's face it—we've been counting calories for decades and it is not working well. Not all calories are created equal. Nutrient-rich foods (natural, unprocessed) are the way to go. Otherwise, as an example, if you consume the "empty" (nonhelpful) calories from sugars, it can make you stay in a state of insulin resistance and challenge your weight management efforts.

of your daily calories should come from fat. Eat no more than 7% of your total calories from saturated fat (for someone on a 2,000-calorie-a-day meal plan, that's 15 grams of saturated fat per day.) A low-calorie choice has 40 calories or fewer per serving, a moderate-calorie choice has 100 calories per serving, and a high-calorie choice has 400 calories or more per serving.

4. **Total fat, cholesterol, and sodium.** These affect your heart health. Consider the following:
   - The overall amount of fat is important to note but not all fat is created equal. Unsaturated fats are heart healthy; trans fats are not and should be avoided.
   - The goal for cholesterol consumption is less than 300 milligrams per day, and for those with cardiovascular risk, less than 200 milligrams per day.
   - The goal for sodium consumption is less than 2,300 milligrams per day. Foods with 5% or less of recommended daily sodium are low in sodium. Try to select foods that provide 5% or less for sodium per serving (or 140 milligrams sodium per serving). Anything with 20% or more sodium is considered high sodium.

5. **Eyeball protein and check ingredients.** Take a look at the amount of protein in the food you're evaluating and then move on to the ingredient list. Ingredients are listed in order by weight. It's likely that you won't recognize a lot of the ingredients or know what they are. Some items are vague:
   - **Hidden fat**—hydrogenated, oil, and shortening
   - **Hidden sugar**—corn syrup, dextrose, fructose, honey, juice concentrate, lactose, molasses, sucrose, and sugar alcohol
   - **Fat substitutes**—cellulose, dextrin, emulsifier, fiber, gum, polydextrose, maltodextrin, modified food starch, olean, olestra, simplesse, and starch
   - **Sugar substitutes (do not contain calories or carbohydrates)**—Rebaudioside A (Reb A, a purified form of Stevia), acesulfame K, aspartame (NutraSweet or Equal), neotame, saccharin (Sweet'N Low), acesulfame potassium (Sunett), and sucralose (Splenda).

6. **Glance at the percent (%) daily value.** This gives you an idea of the nutrient value, based on a 2,000-calorie diet. This information is helpful when considering the nutrients you want to get more of, like calcium and potassium, and vitamin

content that adds up to the 100% recommended daily value.

- 20% or more is a rich source
- 10–19% is a good source
- less than 5% is a low source (good choice for fats, not a good choice for calcium)

Give it a try

Compare these labels for a popular cookie. Which one would you choose?

Cookie baked with 100% whole grain:

Nutrition Facts
Serving Size 3 Cookies (33g)
Servings Per Container About 14

Amount Per Serving

Calories 150   Calories from Fat 70

	% Daily Value*
Total Fat 8g	12%
Saturated Fat 2.5g	13%
Trans Fat 0g	
Polyunsaturated Fat 2.5g	
Monounsaturated Fat 2g	
Cholesterol 0mg	0%
Sodium 110mg	5%
Total Carbohydrate 22g	7%
Dietary Fiber 2g	8%
Sugars 10g	
Protein 2g	

Vitamin A 0%	•	Vitamin C 0%
Calcium 0%	•	Iron 4%

* Percent Daily Values are based on a 2,000 calorie diet. Your daily values may be higher or lower depending on your calorie needs:

	Calories:	2,000	2,500
Total Fat	Less than	65g	80g
Sat Fat	Less than	20g	25g
Cholesterol	Less than	300mg	300mg
Sodium	Less than	2,400mg	2,400mg
Total Carbohydrate		300g	375g
Dietary Fiber		25g	30g

INGREDIENTS: WHOLE GRAIN WHEAT FLOUR, SEMISWEET CHOCOLATE CHIPS (SUGAR, CHOCOLATE, COCOA BUTTER, DEXTROSE, SOY LECITHIN - AN EMULSIFIER), SUGAR, SOYBEAN OIL, PARTIALLY HYDROGENATED COTTONSEED OIL, HIGH FRUCTOSE CORN SYRUP, LEAVENING (BAKING SODA, AMMONIUM PHOSPHATE), SALT, WHEY (FROM MILK), NATURAL AND ARTIFICIAL FLAVOR, CARAMEL COLOR.

Cookie with real chocolate chunks:

Nutrition Facts
Serving Size 1 Cookie (17g)
Servings Per Container About 23

Amount Per Serving

Calories 80   Calories from Fat 40

	% Daily Value*
Total Fat 4.5g	7%
Saturated Fat 1.5g	8%
Trans Fat 0g	
Polyunsaturated Fat 1.5g	
Monounsaturated Fat 1g	
Cholesterol 0mg	0%
Sodium 55mg	2%
Total Carbohydrate 11g	4%
Dietary Fiber Less than 1g	2%
Sugars 6g	
Protein Less than 1g	

Vitamin A 0%	•	Vitamin C 0%
Calcium 0%	•	Iron 2%

* Percent Daily Values are based on a 2,000 calorie diet. Your daily values may be higher or lower depending on your calorie needs:

	Calories:	2,000	2,500
Total Fat	Less than	65g	80g
Sat Fat	Less than	20g	25g
Cholesterol	Less than	300mg	300mg
Sodium	Less than	2,400mg	2,400mg
Total Carbohydrate		300g	375g
Dietary Fiber		25g	30g

INGREDIENTS: ENRICHED FLOUR (WHEAT FLOUR, NIACIN, REDUCED IRON, THIAMINE MONONITRATE (VITAMIN B1), RIBOFLAVIN (VITAMIN B2), FOLIC ACID), SEMISWEET CHOCOLATE CHUNKS (SUGAR, CHOCOLATE, DEXTROSE, COCOA BUTTER, MILKFAT, SOY LECITHIN - AN EMULSIFIER, SALT, VANILLA), SUGAR, SOYBEAN OIL, SEMISWEET CHOCOLATE CHIPS (SUGAR, CHOCOLATE, COCOA BUTTER, DEXTROSE, SOY LECITHIN - AN EMULSIFIER), PARTIALLY HYDROGENATED COTTONSEED OIL, FRUCTOSE, LEAVENING (BAKING SODA, AMMONIUM PHOSPHATE), SALT, MOLASSES, HIGH FRUCTOSE CORN SYRUP, WHEY (FROM MILK), SOY LECITHIN (EMULSIFIER), ARTIFICIAL FLAVOR, CARAMEL COLOR.

Which cookie is better? It's not so clear. The serving size is three of the "healthier" whole-grain cookies, which have twice the calories, carbs, and fat as one regular cookie with real chocolate chunks. If you were able to eat just one of the cookies with chocolate chunks, the taste is better and you'd be better off. Unless you have incredible restraint, however, most people cannot eat just one cookie.

The intent of this exercise is to get you thinking about options, not to encourage you to run down to the store and load up on cookies or sweets! You may be struggling with how to shift eating patterns that have included regular consumption of desserts. This exercise was meant to open up a conversation about the way advertising can mislead you, about how there are no forbidden foods, and about the fact that quality and quantity are paramount with diabetes self-management, as is personal satisfaction with the dining experience. Your registered dietitian (RD) can give you tools to help you *enjoy* your food and navigate ways to incorporate an occasional treat into a balanced diet plan.

The following summary compares vanilla-flavored Yoplait yogurts.

Type	Original	Light Thick and Creamy	Whips!	Light
Serving size	6 ounces	6 ounces	6 ounces	6 ounces
Total carbohydrates (grams)	33	31	25	16
Calories	170	180	160	100
Total fat grams	1.5	2.5	4	0
Saturated fat grams	1	1.5	2.5	0

Which one would you choose? The light version has the least carbohydrate and fat, so why not try a light flavor on your next trip to the grocery store?

Comparing Nutrition Facts labels is a lifetime worth of discovery. This is just a simple overview to get you pointed in the right direction. Don't let that Nutrition Facts label intimidate you! With a little time and perseverance, you'll get the hang of this very helpful tool.

The Nutrition Facts label claim to fame

You'll often see eye-catching advertisements on food packages, such as "low fat" or "healthy." Do you really know what you are about to consume? These are government-approved definitions for claims made on food labels, but what do they mean? First off, remember that all of them are based on *one serving*.

Nutrition Facts Label Definitions

Calorie-free: less than 5 calories per serving

Cholesterol-free: less than 2 milligrams cholesterol per 50-gram serving of food

Extra lean: less than 5% total fat, 2 or fewer grams of saturated fat, and less than 95 milligrams cholesterol

Fat-free: less than 0.5 gram of fat

Fewer: (whether altered or not) 25% less of a nutrient or calories than a similar-referenced product (e.g., one brand can have 25% less sodium than another)

Healthy: low in fat and saturated fat and has limited amounts of cholesterol and sodium. Single food items must also contain at least 10% of one or more of the following: vitamin A or C, iron, calcium, protein, or fiber. Sodium should be less than 480 milligrams per serving and less than 600 milligrams per serving for entrées.

Lean: less than 10% total fat, 4.5 or fewer grams of saturated fat, and less than 95 milligrams cholesterol

Less: see *Fewer*

Less sodium: at least 25% less sodium than the regular product (but not necessarily low in sodium)

Low calorie: 40 calories or less per serving

Low cholesterol: less than 20 milligrams cholesterol per 50 grams serving

Low fat: 3 grams of fat or less

Low saturated fat: 1 gram of saturated fat or less

Low sodium: 140 milligrams of sodium or less

Light or "lite": one-third fewer calories or half the fat of the reference food; may also describe product's texture and color

No added salt: no salt added to the product during processing

Organic: grown or raised without synthetic fertilizers, pesticides, or hormones in a way to enhance the ecological balance of natural systems

Reduced: nutritionally altered product with at least 25% less of a nutrient or calories than the regular product

Salt-free or sodium-free: less than 5 milligrams of sodium

Sugar-free: less than 0.5 gram of sugar

Unsalted: see *No added salt*

Very low sodium: 35 milligrams of sodium or less

PERSONAL GOAL

Date: _____ I will:

Enter my weight:_____

☐ When I am about to choose a food, ask myself, "Is that a carb, protein, or fat?"

☐ Get a carbohydrate-counting resource (check www.diabetes.org or www.dlife.com, or visit your local bookstore or library).

☐ Experiment with favorite foods and dishes. Test glucose before and 2 hours after that meal. Record my results for further analysis in next week's section.

☐ Read at least one food label (Nutrition Facts label) a day, paying attention to the portion size and carbohydrates.

☐ Put Nutrition Facts labels on the back burner for now and instead freeze some grapes for a fun snack (10–15 grapes is the serving size for approximately 15 grams of carbohydrate).

☐ Use the Food and Activity Diary to write down everything I eat for the next week.

☐ Measure out 1 cup of cooked rice to visualize what 45 grams of carbohydrate looks like.

☐ Find a local RD who can help me with an individualized plan.

☐ Other: _____.

 Are you on a good label or a bad label?

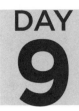

DAY
9

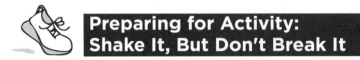

**Preparing for Activity:
Shake It, But Don't Break It**

Why do I need to take precautions before exercising?

You want to ensure that your system can tolerate increased activity without doing any harm. If you have risk factors for coronary artery disease, such as high blood pressure, high cholesterol, early signs of kidney changes (as evidenced by a urine test that shows positive for albuminuria—explained further on Day 27), or a family history of heart disease at a young age, then consider the following:

1. Start with low-intensity exercise and increase the intensity and duration slowly, and
2. Ask your health-care provider about any special precautions you need to take with your exercise program.

Special mention about blood pressure

Diabetes is associated with heart disease and high blood pressure, so it is important to know your risk. What is your blood pressure? If it's uncontrolled with results consistently higher than the target of 140/80 mmHg, ask your health-care provider which exercises are appropriate and safe for you to do.

I don't like the look of comfortable shoes

Comfortable, stylish shoes are available, and it is a shame to have to look so hard to find them. Women's shoes are the worst. Who are these designers? Proper foot attire can prevent a host of problems. If your shoes don't fit, you'll be at risk for blisters, and if those blisters break open, you'll be at risk for infection, pain, and falls. If your feet tend to swell, shop for shoes at the end of the day. Select shoes with cushioned soles and that allow room for your toes to wiggle. Wear cotton or seamless, breathable socks that don't squeeze your ankles or legs like a rubber band.

We take our feet for granted until something goes wrong. All it takes is a foot injury or a fall to make us notice their importance. Treat your feet like royalty. Diabetes that is not controlled for months and years can cause a loss of sensation in the feet due to nerve damage (neuropathy). Small foot problems can turn into big ones. People generally hear about the horrors of amputation and ulcers. It's one of the first things people mention when getting diagnosed, "I don't want to lose a leg." Of course not! With precautions, you can protect your feet for a lifetime. Do you think that you already have a foot problem? Call a podiatrist and make an appointment now!

What Makes a Good, Comfortable Shoe?

1. Support (you shouldn't be able to fold the shoe in two or wring it out like a towel!)
2. Cushion (you shouldn't feel the earth move under your feet)
3. Seamless across the toes (to prevent blisters)
4. Space to wiggle your toes

You can check with your healthcare provider about local vendors, and you can check out these companies that offer many stylish shoes for people with diabetes:
- Therapeutic Footwear at www. phc-online.com, click on Footwear & Accessories (866-772-4581).
- Footwear for a healthier you with ACOR at store.acor.com (800-237-2267).
- For feet in need of special care, go to Drew Shoes at www.drewshoe. com (800-837-3739).

Safety tips while walking

Besides having the right kind of shoes, be aware of your surroundings. We belong to an iPod nation and are glued to our cell phones, so turn down the volume and look around at what you're walking into. Street crime and unsafe neighborhoods can keep us inside, but with a little planning, a healthy walk is not out of the question. Walk with a buddy. Plan your walking route to promote your personal safety. Keep an eye out for those poorly maintained sidewalks.

Foot Care Tips

•Clean your feet daily with mild soap and water.

•Dry thoroughly, especially between the toes.

•Apply lotion to your heels but not in between toes.

•Trim nails straight across and file the corners with an emery board.

•Avoid soaking just your feet (this actually dries out the skin and increases the risk of infection).

•Don't use any sharp objects on your feet (such as razor blades) or anything that could make them bleed (pumice stones).

•Avoid tight-fitting socks, nylons, or shoes.

•Check your shoes for any debris or other unwanted objects.

•Treat any cuts or scrapes right away with warm water and soap, apply a thin layer of antibiotic ointment, cover loosely with a bandage, and try to stay off your feet.

•Look for color changes, redness, tenderness, swelling, and ingrown toenails.

•Notify your doctor if any blisters do not heal within a couple of days.

•Get professional treatment for corns and calluses (don't use over-the-counter chemical corn/wart removers).

•Don't use heating pads or hot water bottles on your feet.

•Avoid crossing your legs (cuts off circulation).

•Do foot exercises and stretches.

What about pedicures?

They sure feel great, but pedicures generally are not recommended for people with diabetes because of the risk for infection. Very few pedicure establishments are ever inspected, and standards do not exist. If this brings you pleasure that you cannot live without, minimize your risk by purchasing and brining your own pedicure instruments, make sure you see the tub lined with new plastic before you get in it, and don't let them cut too close or get too vigorous with your cuticles. All it takes is one little nick of the skin and you can get a fungal infection that can take months to cure. Tell them you have diabetes, to keep water temperature to 95°F, to avoid razors, and to be gentle. And if you shave your legs, do not do so for 2 days before the appointment to decrease your chance of infection. You can also see a foot care specialist or podiatrist for difficult-to-trim nails.

PERSONAL GOAL

Date: _____ I will:

☐ Ask my health-care provider if my blood pressure is safe for me to exercise.

☐ Slow down if I get out of breath or can't talk freely while exercising.

☐ Snack if my glucose is less than 100 before exercising (1/2 fruit or 1/2 sandwich) and bring glucose tablets with me if I take diabetes pills or insulin.

☐ Do a shoe turnaround (so that your closet has only comfortable pairs).

☐ Wear shoes or slippers at home (which is where most foot injuries occur).

☐ Remove socks and shoes whenever I see my health-care provider.

☐ Put lotion on my feet every day, except between the toes (some lotion is better than none; look for nonfragrance types with deep moisturizing qualities).

☐ Ask my partner for a foot rub (and give one in return)!

☐ Wear a stylish business suit with comfortable shoes.

☐ Other: _____.

 I treat my feet like royalty.
So where's the paparazzi?

DAY 10

Glucose Quantum Leaps

How low is low? What is hypoglycemia?

Hypoglycemia is the technical name for low blood glucose when readings are less than 70 mg/dL. Causes include too much medication, too little food, increased exercise without adjustments to medication, and alcohol intake. If you have more than two hypoglycemic events in 1 week, report it to your health-care provider.

Treatment of hypoglycemia.

If your blood glucose is low, you need sugar and *fast*. Follow the **Rule of 15**:

If your blood glucose is less than 70 mg/dL, take 15 grams of carbohydrate (*choose one*: 4 glucose tablets, 4 ounces of juice, 8 ounces of milk, 4 teaspoons of sugar, 1/4 cup of regular soda, or a small box of raisins) and wait 15 minutes. That's the hard part. Recheck blood glucose level. If it is still less than 70 mg/dL, take another 15 grams of carbohydrate, wait, and check again in 15 minutes. Once blood glucose rises to more than 70 mg/dL, have a small snack (or if it is close to mealtime, eat your meal).

Even better, follow the Rule of Playing It Safe. If you are on a medication that makes your pancreas release more insulin (see Day 12 for a list), carry quick-acting glucose with you at all times (see previous examples). It can save your life. Also, if you happen to be without your monitor and suspect you are running low, when in doubt, treat for low blood glucose. If left untreated, it can lead to coma and death. Take the time

> ### Symptoms of Hypoglycemia
> Irritability, shakiness, sweating, dizziness, rapid heartbeat, profound hunger (the "mean, get-out-of-my-way" type of hunger), blurred vision, weakness, drowsiness, and difficulty walking or talking. Sometimes there are few or no symptoms.

to get some form of medical identification that will help in the event of an emergency, such as a medical alert bracelet, necklace, or wallet card.

How high is high? What is hyperglycemia?

The technical name for glucose levels more than 200 mg/dL is hyperglycemia. It can be caused by too much food, too little exercise, not enough medicine or insulin, stress, injury, or illness.

Treatment of hyperglycemia

Treating hyperglycemia depends on the underlying cause. Hydration helps to dilute the high readings to a small extent, so drink some water; take additional medication, if your physician has authorized you to do so; and light exercise might help if your reading is due to consuming too many carbohydrates. Continue checking glucose a few times a day until the values come back down.

Consistent readings more than 250 mg/dL should be reported to your health-care provider. In extreme cases, hyperglycemia can lead to coma. Scary, yes, but preventable with monitoring and calls to your health-care team.

Symptoms of Hyperglycemia

Feeling sleepy after eating, excessive thirst, overall tiredness, blurred vision, and frequent urination (especially in the middle of the night). Sometimes there are no symptoms.

Update on Glucose Results

Review your blood glucose results from the past week. Which meals had a less than 50 mg/dL increase from before to 2 hours after the meal? Make a mental note so you will feel more comfortable having those meals. For the ones that increased more than 50 points, experiment with the same meal but move some of the carbohydrate to a snack and load up on veggies or increase the protein content to assess how your blood glucose will respond.

PERSONAL GOAL

Date: _____ I will:

☐ Keep an organized record of glucose values and a list of any comments and questions to bring to my next medical appointment.

☐ Test my glucose more often if I am under the weather, don't feel well for any reason, or have had a change in medicine.

☐ Call my health-care provider when my glucose patterns do not make sense.

☐ Ask to see a diabetes specialist (an endocrinologist) to help stabilize my diabetes (check the American Association of Clinical Endocrinologists website at www.aace.com/resources/find-an-endocrinologist to find one locally).

☐ Make a commitment to test my glucose for as long as I have the gift of life.

☐ Give myself a minibreak from testing only when my glucose is stable and I feel great.

☐ Check my glucose at different times (such as 2 hours after lunch or dinner or after exercise).

☐ Test less when more than half of my glucose values are in target range for a particular time.

☐ Call my health-care provider for two or more readings less than 70 mg/dL or more than 250 mg/dL.

☐ Other: _____.

After analyzing these glucose trends, I'm ready to predict the weather.

DAY 11

Medication Literacy

What does literacy have to do with diabetes self-management? If you can read and understand health information, then you are more likely to take your medications correctly and have a better chance at controlling your diabetes. But there's more to it than that, such as navigating medication adjustments, counting carbs, and understanding how to respond to blood glucose levels.

Do you know what this wording means? "Take one tablet daily for 7 days, then two tablets twice a day." For the first 7 days, you take only one tablet a day. After day 7, you will take two pills at a time, two times a day, probably in the morning and evening. It's a short sentence, but there's a lot of important information there.

Avoid mistakes when you receive a prescription; ask your healthcare provider and pharmacist about how to take the drug.

Know Your Medications

Ask these questions whenever you receive a medication.

What does this drug do?
Why am I taking this drug?
When do I take it?
Do I take it with food?
How much do I take?
What should I do if I miss a dose?
How long will I be taking this drug?
Will it interact with my other medications?
What are common side effects?

PERSONAL GOAL

Date: _____ I will:

☐ Put all of my medications in a bag and review them with my pharmacist or health-care provider.

☐ Go through all my medication bottles and prescriptions and throw away any I'm not using or that have expired. Check www.fda.gov and search "safe disposal of medications" for instructions on the best way to do this, or ask my pharmacist.

☐ Go over all of my medication names, doses, frequency, purposes, and side effects, including over-the-counter drugs, vitamins, and herbal remedies. Make a chart with this information, so it is easily available and so I can check generic names to avoid duplication.

☐ Be able to recognize my medications by shape, color, size, and name.

☐ Other: _____.

 Researchers are trying to find someone who only eats 1/2 cup of ice cream every other day.

DAY
12

 Sidestepping Side Effects

Many unpleasant side effects of medications can be prevented. For example, some medications need to be taken with meals; others should be taken on an empty stomach. Check the chart beginning on the next page for some common oral and non-insulin injectable medicines, their possible side effects, and ways to avoid them. This is a summary. For detailed information pertaining to the type of diabetes medication you may be taking, check the index as several of these have more information in subsequent chapters (e.g., insulin).

ORAL MEDICATIONS

Type of oral diabetes medicine (how it works)	Brand name (generic name)	Dosage	Timing	Possible side effects or issues
Insulin secretagogues (make the pancreas release more insulin)	Amaryl (glimepride)	1–2 mg per day; max 8 milligrams	Before the first meal	Hypoglycemia (see Day 10).
	Glucotrol (glipizide)	5 milligrams	30 minutes before the first meal	
		40 milligrams max, divided	30 minutes before breakfast and dinner	
	Glucotrol XL (extended release glipizide)	2.5–20 milligrams per day	Before the first meal	Hypoglycemia. Do not crush or break pill in two.
	Glynase PresTab (glyburide)	1.5, 3, and 6 milligrams; max 12 milligrams per day	Before the first meal; second dose may be taken before dinner	Hypoglycemia.
	Micronase (glyburide)	2.5 or 5 milligrams per day	Before the first meal	Risk for prolonged hypoglycemia in people with kidney problems or the elderly.
		max of 20 milligrams, divided	Before breakfast and dinner	
	Prandin (repaglinide)	0.5–2 milligrams	Just before meals	Do not take if you skip a meal.
	Starlix (nateglinide)	60 or 120 milligrams	Three times daily, before meals	

Type of oral diabetes medicine (how it works)	Brand name (generic name)	Dosage	Timing	Possible side effects or issues
Biguanides (limit glucose production from the liver)	Glucophage (metformin)	500–2,500 milligrams	Once or twice daily with food	Bloating, gas, and diarrhea can be minimized by taking it after a meal and building up tolerance to medication slowly (1 pill a day with large meal for 1 week before adding a second pill in the morning). Avoid use if you have kidney, liver, or heart disease or if you are elderly. Stop before having surgery or taking X-rays.
	Glumetza (once-a-day, extended release metformin)			
Thiazolidine-diones or TZDs (reduce the body's resistance to insulin)	Actos (pioglitazone)	15–45 milligrams per day	With or without food	Can cause swelling of the ankles. Not recommended with congestive heart failure. Liver tests needed. Can take 6 weeks to reach full effect.
Alpha-glucosidase inhibitors (slow the absorption of carbohydrates in the intestines)	Precose (acarbose)	25–300 milligrams	With first bite of a meal, up to three times a day	Abdominal pain, gas, and diarrhea. If used with insulin or insulin secretagogues, hypoglycemia must be treated with pure glucose (tabs or gel) as Precose can interfere with the absorption of other carbohydrates.
	Glyset (miglitol)	50–300 milligrams		

Type of oral diabetes medicine (how it works)	Brand name (generic name)	Dosage	Timing	Possible side effects or issues
DPP-4 inhibitors (increase insulin secretion only when glucose is high)	Januvia (sitagliptin)	25–100 milligrams	Around the same time of day, regardless of mealtime	When used with secretagogues or insulin, a lower dose of secretagogues or insulin may be required to minimize the risk of hypoglycemia.
	Onglyza (saxagliptin)	2.5 or 5 milligrams		
	Tradjenta (linagliptin)	5 milligrams		
SGLT2 inhibitors (increase the amount of glucose leaving the body in the urine and delay glucose absorption in the intestines)	Invokana (canagliflozin)	100 or 300 milligrams	Once daily before the first meal of the day	Has been shown to reduce systolic blood pressure, cholesterol, and weight. Slight risk for urinary tract infection or genital fungal infection. If taking insulin, plan on reducing dose.
	Forxiga (dapagliflozin)	5 or 10 milligrams		
Dopamine agonist (keeps the liver from releasing too much glucose; improves muscle sensitivity to insulin)	Cycloset (bromocriptine mesylate)	0.8 milligrams daily, increase weekly by one tablet until 1.6–4.8 milligrams is reached	Within 2 hours of waking up in the morning with food	Nausea common at first; slowly increase dose as directed. May cause headache; do not use with certain migraine medications

Note: Several types of combination medications are available (two types of medication in one pill). Common ones include Glucovance (glyburide/metformin), Metaglip (glipizide/metformin), and Janumet (sitagliptin/metformin). Ask your pharmacist or health-care provider if any of yours are available in combination form.

INJECTABLE MEDICATIONS

Type of injectable (and how it works)	Brand name (generic name)	Dosage	Timing	Possible side effects or issues
Incretin Mimetic GLP-1 Analogs (glucagon-like peptide 1 agonists) Stimulate pancreas to produce insulin when blood glucose is high. Slow stomach emptying. Decrease appetite. Decrease glucagon release after meals.	Byetta (exenatide)	5–10 micrograms	Within 1 hour before morning and evening meals	Nausea common at first. Vomiting, dizziness, and headache may occur. Hypoglycemia if a risk if taken with pills listed under secretagogue. Byetta: do not take if you skip a meal; do not take after the meal as it may cause vomiting. Byetta is not recommended for people with severe kidney problems, high triglycerides, or digestion problems. Bydureon must be injected immediately after the powder is mixed.
	Bydureon (exenatide extended release)	2 milligrams	Once every 7 days (weekly), at any time of the day and with or without meals	
	Victoza (liraglutide)	Start with 0.6 milligrams daily for 1 week; if ineffective increase to 1.2 milligrams for 1 week; if ineffective increase to 1.8 milligrams	Once a day with or without food	
Amylino-mimetics Mimic a hormone that is normally cosecreted with insulin. Slow stomach emptying. Decrease appetite. Decrease glucagon release after meals.	Symlin (pramlintide acetate)	15–120 micrograms	Just before meals, up to three times a day	For type 1 and 2 diabetes. Reduce short-acting, mealtime insulin by 50% when starting Symlin to prevent hypoglycemia . Don't mix in same syringe with insulin. Nausea and vomiting are common at first. Not recommended for people with digestive problems.

Note: Insulin is covered in detail in Month 6.

PERSONAL GOAL

Date: _____ I will:

☐ Find out whether I take my pills before or after I eat.
☐ Tell my health-care provider about any possible side effects (nausea, lows, swollen feet).
☐ Talk with my health-care provider before stopping medications or changing doses, or ask for a plan on how to adjust the dose.
☐ Keep my medicines in a temperature-controlled environment (avoid heat extremes).
☐ Check the expiration dates on my medicines.
☐ Be adventurous and read the package insert.
☐ Find out if I need to stop taking metformin before an X-ray or surgery.
☐ Other: _____.

 The only side effect I feel from these medications is in my wallet.

DAY
13

Be Astute with Veggies and Fruit

Flourish with Fruit

I was told to cut out fruit because it makes my blood glucose go up.

Eliminate an entire, nutritious food group? No! Science proves that fruits are an integral part of healthy eating. Like all other food groups that contain carbohydrate, fruits raise your glucose level, but they are also rich in fiber, vitamins, minerals, and phytochemicals, which act as antioxidants to protect the cells in your body. They do pack a carb punch, so you need to know how much to eat.

Is fruit a good snack choice?

Yes! Choose from fresh, frozen, canned (with light syrup, packed in its own juice or water), or dried fruit. If you must drink juice, try diluting it with water (unless you are using it to treat a low blood glucose, as reviewed on Day 10) or keep your portion to 4 ounces.

What's a serving size of fruit?

Visualize your cupped hand filled with fruit. That is one serving size. Examples include one small piece of fresh fruit; 1/2 cup of fresh, canned, or frozen fruit; 1/4 cup dried fruit; or 4 ounces of juice. Current recommendations suggest that people with diabetes should eat two to four servings of fruit a day, not eaten all at once. This is individualized, based on your age, sex, and level of physical activity. Do you enjoy a whole bowl of cherries or tall glasses of orange juice?

Making choices like these can send your blood glucose into outer space. Think about how many oranges are needed to get 4 ounces of juice. You'll end up with the sugar content of several oranges just from one glass.

Be Vibrant with Veggies

If you are trying to lower glucose, cholesterol, or blood pressure or to lose or maintain weight, vegetables will help. Veggies are low in calories, low in carbohydrate, and high in fiber. Nonstarchy vegetables can be eaten in larger quantities without affecting glucose much at all. Find ways to enjoy them: zucchini, broccoli, spinach, red bell peppers, and, yes, even sweet potatoes. How about giving your veggies a little extra punch with vegetable broth and dried spices (oregano or Italian seasonings)? There are so many fun, seasonal, flavorful veggies available (the following chart gives you some ideas). If you don't like one, try another, and another.

What's a serving size of veggies?

Cup both hands in front of you. That's the recommended portion size for uncooked vegetables (1 cup), the largest serving size of any food group. For cooked veggies, the serving size is 1/2 cup. MyPlate recommends that most adults eat the following each week: at least 3 cups of leafy green vegetables, at least 2 cups of orange vegetables, and at least 3 cups of dry beans and peas. Pile up on the nonstarchy ones. In looking at the following chart, how many different types of veggies have you consumed this past week? How were they prepared? Get creative in finding ways to incorporate more green in your life.

Dark green	Orange	Other	Starchy veggies, dry beans and peas (contain carbohydrate)
Bok choy	Acorn squash	Artichokes	Corn
Broccoli	Butternut squash	Asparagus	Black beans
Collard greens	Carrots	Bean sprouts	Black-eyed peas
Dark green leafy lettuce	Pumpkin	Beets	Garbanzo beans
Kale	Sweet potatoes	Brussels sprouts	Green lima beans
Romaine lettuce		Cabbage	Green peas
Spinach		Cauliflower	Kidney beans
Swiss chard		Celery	Lentils
Turnip greens		Cucumbers	Lima beans
Watercress		Eggplant	Navy beans
		Green beans	Pinto beans
		Green or red bell peppers	Potatoes
		Iceberg lettuce	Soy beans
		Mushrooms	Split peas
		Okra	Tofu
		Onions	White beans
		Parsnips	
		Tomatoes	
		Turnips	
		Wax beans	
		Zucchini	

What is a starchy vegetable?

Starchy veggies are those that contain more carbohydrate, such as peas, corn, potatoes, yams, and sweet potatoes. You can certainly eat these; just know to factor in their carb count or balance them out with protein choices.

What about dried beans?

Dried beans provide protein and are a source of starch. They are good for you but do consider their carb content in your meal planning.

Revolutionary Idea

As promised, topics are presented in an order to have the biggest impact in helping you to manage diabetes. Time to plant a seed: a plant-based diet.

Many people want a nonmedication solution to diabetes and its associated issues. Coined "Food as Medicine" by Dr. Neal Barnard, a vegan diet can sometimes improve type 2 diabetes by setting aside animal products and keeping oils to a minimum. This may seem radical. It depends on what is "radical" in your book. Wouldn't it be outrageous to feel great, maximize your diabetes health, limit the amount of medications needed, and prevent surgery to repair clogged arteries? We can dig our own grave with a spoon by routinely consuming foods that cause inflammation and are not nutritious (if only they didn't taste so bloody good!). It *is* hard to make the shift to plant-based eating; it requires time to learn and to be inventive as your taste buds adjust to a scrumptious way of eating. You may long for eggs benedict, but what is more important: that breakfast or your health? For many people, the answer will be a fill-in-the-blank meal containing animal products. That's fine. For those who are willing to try a different approach, however, a vegan diet may be your bullet train to health. See Week 19 for further discussion.

Not so radical

Think carefully about the first thing you put on your plate as it usually will take up about 60%. Best to go for the nonstarchy veggies first and load at least half of your plate with them. Also, bigger plates increase overall portions by 36%. Is it time for new dishes?

PERSONAL GOAL

Date: _____ I will:

☐ Check how much fruit and veggies I need to have at www.cdc.gov/nutrition/everyone/fruitsvegetables/howmany.html.
☐ Eat fruit rather than drink it.
☐ Help out my sweet tooth by giving it fruit rather than candy.
☐ Try a new vegetable.
☐ Start adding a serving of vegetables to dinner 2–3 days a week and work up to covering half of my plate with veggies at most dinners.
☐ Pay for the convenience of prewashed, precut veggies (cuts down on prep time).
☐ Chop up veggie slices and have them ready in the fridge for a healthy snack.
☐ Get yummy plant-based recipe ideas with this 21-day vegan kick-start program from Physicians Committee for Responsible Medicine pcrm.org/kickstartHome/index.cfm.
☐ Download and read this vegetarian starter kit to inspire my options pcrm.org/health/diets/vsk/vegetarian-starter-kit.
☐ Other: _____.

Veggies are my friends. I really should see them more often.

DAY 14

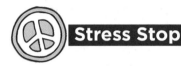

Stress Stop

To stress or not to stress

You've been dealing with the stress of diabetes and no doubt trying not to obsess about all the details. What are *other* sources of stress in your life? (See the section "Diabetes Dollars and Sense.") How do you respond? How can you limit, prevent or resolve them?

Positive Ways I Can Cope with My Diabetes and Manage Overall Stress

Circle one item from the below to be your focus for the week.

- Tell my family and friends about ways in which they can help.
- Be patient with myself.
- Shift my perspective.
- Take a different route to work or home.
- Get out and enjoy nature.
- Go for a 10-minute walk.
- Listen to the birds.
- Avoid negative people.
- Read for pleasure.
- Acknowledge my level of stress: accept to stay there or change it.
- Celebrate life.
- Find humor every day.
- Pick my battles.
- Keep writing in my journal.
- Do something different.
- Look forward rather than backward.
- Know my limits.
- Get enough rest and sleep regularly.
- Daydream.

One strategy is to focus on things you *can* change, such as choosing with whom to share your energy, what you eat, when you exercise, how you react, how you communicate your needs, how many items you put on your to-do list, and how much time you spend on any given task. Focusing on things you can't change will only add to your stress level. You can't change other people, your upbringing, your age, number of hours in a day, a long wait for a scheduled appointment, an accident, or a death in the family.

Given the proper tools and practice, you can self-regulate stress. Imagine a life of being able to effectively handle the stress that gets thrown in your lap. According to Laurel Mellin, the founder of Emotional Brain Training, 80% of disease is caused by stress. Stress causes a cascade of hormones, such as cortisol, which in turn raises insulin resistance. Find ways to mitigate it on a daily basis.

Diabetes Dollars and Sense: How to Pay Less and Reduce Your Stress

Do you feel like diabetes already stole your favorite dessert and now, your paycheck, too?

Let's be frank: Diabetes self-care is expensive and that can add a lot of stress to your daily life. Medical expenditures and out-of-pocket costs are higher for people with diabetes than for those without diabetes.

Tips on saving your health-care bucks

At home

- Get friendly with your health insurance company. Find out exactly what is covered: from medications to test strips to co-pays for medical visits and diabetes classes.
- Look for coupons in diabetes magazines or incentives through diabetes supply manufacturers' literature and websites.
- Check for local programs that provide health care or supplies to individuals in need (the diabetes program or medical social worker at your local hospital will have the most knowledge about these resources).
- Take the time to research the programs from pharmaceutical

companies that offer free drugs to people in need.

- Review your medical bills for accuracy, and don't be shy to ask for itemized explanations. You may catch expensive errors. Keep notes (details of dates, times, contact person, what was said) and follow-up.

At the health-care provider's office

- Discuss the burden of out-of-pocket costs.
- Ask for coupons, samples of your medication (especially if this is a new drug you are just trying out), or test strips. Some offices are lucky enough to get test strip samples. Coupons are not valid with government insurance (Medicare, Medicaid, and Tricare).
- Ask if you can switch to generic versions of any prescriptions as they cost less than brand-name drugs.
- Find out whether your medications come in a combination form.
- Bring a list of medications covered by your insurance provider, also known as a formulary. The list of prescription drugs in this formulary encourages enrollees to select lower-cost drugs. Ask your provider whether switching over to equivalent medicines listed on your formulary would work for your situation.
- If you take insulin, ask which insulin and delivery system will save you money. Some plans cover insulin pens at the same co-pay.
- Make an appointment with the social worker (usually there's one affiliated with your clinic; if not, go to a local community center or look online). She or he may be able to find out if you can get new or improved insurance through your employer, a family member, or a state or federal program.

At the pharmacy

- Shop around, especially for test strips and syringes or pen needles, which tend to cost less at bigger chain pharmacies in your area.
- Ask whether a 90-day supply of prescriptions would be less expensive.

On the Internet

- Avoid scams. Watch out for fake products that promise you the moon. Visit the Food and Drug Administration (FDA) website (www.fda.gov) and search "scams" or "health fraud" for more details.

- Check in with prescription assistance programs. They provide free or nearly free medications to those who qualify. Typically, to qualify you must be a U.S. resident, have an income level below the poverty line, and not have prescription medication insurance. The best way to find out if you qualify is to contact one of these programs: The Partnership for Prescription Assistance (www.pparx.org or call 1-877-477-2669), Rx Outreach (www.rxoutreach.org or call 1-800-769-3880), or SelectCare Benefits Network (www.myrxadvocate.com or call 1-877-331-0362).

At work

- Sign up for a flexible spending account that allows you to use pretax dollars for your health-care costs.
- Before leaving a job, talk to the human resources staff about purchasing extended health insurance through the Consolidated Omnibus Budget Reconciliation Act (COBRA) or ask about other options.

What about Medicare and Medicaid?

Medicare is a federal program that provides health coverage for people more than 65 years of age, those who are disabled, and those with kidney failure. To learn more about Medicare benefits, call the National Diabetes Education Program at 1-800-438-5383 and ask for a copy of "The Power Is in Your Hands" and "Expanded Medicare Coverage of Diabetes Services."

Medicaid is a state government program that provides health insurance for qualified individuals in need. Programs differ among states. Check the local listings to get in contact with your local office.

What if I don't have insurance?

If you don't have insurance, contact the Bureau of Primary Health Care, a service of the Health Resources and Service Administration, to find local health centers that offer health care regardless of your ability to pay, by calling 1-877-464-4772 or visit their website at www.bphc.

hrsa.gov. The American Diabetes Association also has lists of local options and can be reached at 1-800-DIABETES (800-342-2383).

PERSONAL GOAL

Date: _____ I will:

☐ Discuss the costs of diabetes with my health-care provider.
☐ Start a flexible spending account at work so I can use pretax dollars to pay for health-care expenses.
☐ Check out the Partnership for Prescription Assistance at www. pparx.org or call 1-888-662-2669 (they help complete and mail applications ready to sign for you to take to your provider).
☐ Visit another comprehensive resource, www.act1diabetes. org, click on Community Resources, and then select Patient Assistance Programs: The Insider Guide for PWDs (People with Diabetes).
☐ Check out the FDA's website for tips on safely purchasing prescription medications online at www.fda.gov and use the search term "buying medicines over the Internet."
☐ Make a plan to improve my financial health, work to pay off debts, and build up savings.
☐ Before buying something, ask myself whether it will improve my life and move me closer to my goals.
☐ Other: _____.

 Money might not be able to buy happiness, but it can sure buy a lot of test strips.

WEEK 2: REVIEW

Date: _____

What was your track record for meeting your goals during Week 2?

☐ Mostly   ☐ Sometimes   ☐ Rarely
  (80% or more)   (50–80%)   (less than 50%)

Symbol	Related key to diabetes self-management
	Eat wisely
	Be active
	Check numbers (includes glucose/A1C, blood pressure, cholesterol, and weight)
	Reduce stress
	Understand medications
	Solve problems
	Reduce risks
	Add humor

1. Circle the one that was effortless. Focus on your triumphs.
2. Put a question mark next to the one that was troublesome.
   Reflect on ways you might try to tackle obstacles in the week
   to come.

WEEK 3

Laughin' Langerhans

By Theresa Garnero

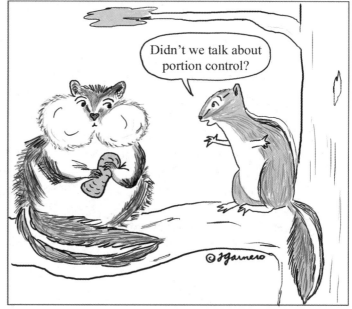

DAY
15

 Let's Go Out to Eat!

How am I supposed to handle going out to eat?

With pleasure and a little preparation. Dining out is meant to be enjoyable, whether it's at a restaurant or at the house of a loved one. Build a plan for success to avoid an awkward situation or unhealthy meal. Here are some tips for satisfying your hunger in a diabetes-friendly way:

Location, location, location. Where you go to eat makes a big difference in whether or not you'll find healthy food choices. Select the restaurant *before* you are hungry! Find ones that allow you healthy options and the ability to substitute menu items. Depending on your menu selection, you might be surprised at how your glucose levels respond.

Discuss your needs. Tell your dinner companions or waiter that you are working on making healthy food choices and ask for their help. You don't have to give them your full medical history to accomplish this. Whom you choose to share the diabetes news with is up to you. It may be helpful, but not essential. You can say, "I'm following a low-carb, low-fat, live-to-be-90 diet."

Be picky. Select baked, grilled, or steamed items. Avoid fried, fatty stuff. Ask for dressings and sauces on the side. Trim off fat and remove skins.

Plan for delays. Delays in getting your food can cause significant problems with hypoglycemia or overeating if you get too hungry. If you know dinner will be late, have some unsalted nuts to stave off the hunger. If you are taking insulin or a medication that causes your pancreas to release more insulin (see Day 12, and review the list of pills under "Insulin secretagogues" in the table Oral Medications), wait until the food is delivered before you take your medicine to prevent hypoglycemia.

Check portions. Serving sizes have increased by up to eight times since the 1970s, and we wonder why our waistlines are expanding! Share a meal or ask for a doggie bag right away, so when the meal arrives, you can put away half to take home instead of being compelled to clean your plate. Definitely share the dessert, on the special occasions it is ordered.

Experiment. Eat at your favorite haunts, and test your glucose levels before the meal and 2 hours after finishing to see how your body handles the meal. If your blood glucose goes up more than 50 mg/dL, try to figure out what happened by going back to the restaurant and trying a slight variation of the original order. Was it a simple case of being starved and wolfing down the entire breadbasket? Or was it a hidden honey teriyaki dressing that did it? Or how about pizza—the gift that keeps on giving? How about other variables, such as stress (getting in an argument, being in pain, fighting a cold)? Sometimes it's not always clear.

Leave room to breathe. Are you in touch with your belly? Do you know the point at which you go from being satisfied to being stuffed?

Is There an Easier Way to Do This?

Yes, there are two popular approaches: Compare serving sizes with everyday objects and follow the Plate Method.

Comparing serving sizes

To get an idea of how much a recommended serving size should be for carbohydrates, protein, and fat, check the following chart and make a mental note. Does this mean that this is all you can have in a day? No. It's a visual guide of building blocks that you can use to add up your carbohydrate intake for a particular meal or snack and give you an idea about what a healthy serving size looks like.

In the Palm of Your Hand

  A palm or a deck of cards is about a medium-sized portion (3 ounces) of meat.

 An open hand is about 2 carbohydrate servings.

 A tennis ball is roughly the size of a medium fruit, 1 cup (45 grams of carb) of cooked pasta, 1 cup (30 grams of carb) of fresh fruit.

 A tight fist means you're good with money and also represents about 1 carbohydrate serving of cooked cereal or ice cream.

 The tip of your thumb is about 1 serving of fat (such as oil or mayonnaise).

 A large egg represents 1/4 cup of raisins.

 or A size C battery or 4 dice is the serving recommendation for low-fat or fat-free cheese.

The Plate Method

Originally described in the Swedish magazine *Van Naring* ("Our Nourishment") in 1970, the Plate Method was adapted by the Idaho Diabetes Care and Education practice group in 1993. Since then, it has helped many individuals with diabetes decide what to eat. Below is a simplistic adaptation to help you get started.

The Plate Method requires basic knowledge about food groups. Not all plates are created equal; that's why it's vital to use a nine-inch plate with this method. Please refer to the special instructions that follow the chart.

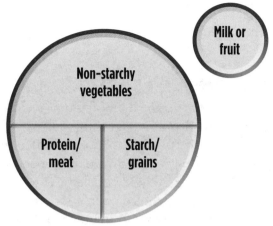

Food Groups and Serving Sizes

Nonstarchy vegetables: Fill half of your plate with one to two servings of nonstarchy vegetables (if you want to have starchy vegetables, such as potatoes, peas, corn, or winter squash, count them as a starch, not vegetables). Examples: 1/2 cup of cooked or 1 cup raw broccoli, spinach, carrots, beets, green beans, cauliflower, zucchini, bell peppers, mushrooms, lettuce, celery, tomato, or cucumber.

Protein/meat or meat substitute: One serving is about 2–4 ounces of fish, lean meat, or skinless chicken and should take up a small portion of the plate (about 1/4). Beans, lentils, or tofu count as 1 carb and 1 lean meat choice. Examples: 3 ounces of white turkey or chicken, tuna (packed in water), halibut, shrimp, scallops, salmon, fat-free cheese, pork, beef, egg (three per week or use an egg substitute), or veggie patties.

Starches/grains: Fill up about 1/4 of the plate. Examples: whole-grain breads (such as 1 slice of whole wheat or rye), a small potato, 1/2 cup pasta, 1/3 cup rice, small bowl of soup or high-fiber cereal, 1/2 English muffin, 1/2 cup of beans, peas, or corn.

Milk: Add an 8-ounce glass of nonfat or low-fat milk. If you don't drink milk, you can add another small serving of carb such as a 6-ounce container of light yogurt or a small roll.

Fruit: Choose one small piece of fruit or a small bowl of berries or melon. Examples: apple, small banana, kiwi, orange, peach;

1 cup raspberries/strawberries, 3/4 cup blueberries, or 15 grapes.

Snacks: Snacks may or may not be needed based on your hunger level, blood glucose levels, and weight loss plans.

How Many Carbs Can I Eat?

Depending on your after-meal blood glucose values and weight-management goals, use this as a beginning guide:

Women: Start with 30–45 grams of carb per meal.

Men: Start with 45–60 grams of carb per meal.

Note: You may hear people refer to a "carb choice" in which 1 carb choice equals 15 grams of carbohydrate (e.g., 1 slice of bread, 1 cup of milk, 1/3 cup of pasta or rice). It is another way to count carbs. In this book, the total grams of carb will be listed.

Of course, the best option is to meet with a registered dietitian first. He or she can get you started on an individualized plan, including how many carbs would be best to meet your needs.

What about Alcohol?

Adding alcohol to diabetes is a big gamble. Diabetes is unpredictable by itself, and alcohol can make blood glucose levels change unpredictably. If you don't drink alcohol, now is not the time to start; wait until your glucose is stable! Much research points to lowering cardiovascular disease risk with moderate alcohol use (no more than 1 drink per day for women, 2 drinks per day for men), but this does not apply to everyone.

Use the following tactics to safely consume alcohol:

- Play it safe, and get your doctor's blessing.
- Check your blood glucose before drinking.
- Have some sort of food with the alcohol (whether it's a meal or some hors d'oeuvres).
- Sip your drinks slowly and consider alternating with water or nonalcoholic drinks.
- Know what constitutes *one* drink (12 ounces of beer, 5 ounces of wine, 1 1/2 ounces of liquor).
- Know *your* limit.
- Alcohol consumed in the evening may cause hypoglycemia up

to 24 hours later, most commonly during the night and after breakfast the next day (especially when combined with after-breakfast exercise).

- Alcohol can reduce your judgment and ability to recognize and react to hypoglycemia.
- Bring supplies for treating hypoglycemia, just to be prepared.
- Limit or avoid sweet alcoholic beverages with fruit juice or high-sugar content.
- Avoid drinking when your diabetes is not well controlled.

Healthy Choices with Ethnic Foods

Do the menus at ethnic restaurants sometimes make it hard to choose the healthiest options? Here are some tips for making healthy choices.

Type	Healthier options	Try to avoid
Chinese	Vegetable dishes; order items for the whole table and share; sauces on the side; low-sodium soy sauce; use chopsticks!	Fried rice; noodles; egg rolls; items described as "crispy," "golden brown," or "sweet and sour"; regular soy sauce
Indian	Chicken tikka masala, shrimp bhuna, fish vindaloo or tandoori-prepared chicken, baked pappadam bread	Fried appetizers; coconut oil; naan; chapatti; roti; ghee (clarified butter); malai (a thick cream)
Italian	Antipasto dish with baked veggies; insalata caprese; share a pasta and salad dish; pasta dishes with a tomato sauce (puttanesca, arrabbiata, vongole); grilled or "griglia"	Garlic bread; bread and butter; pizza (limit yourself to 2 slices and add salad); Alfredo or primavera sauces; items listed as "carbonara," "frito," "saltimbocca," "parmigiana"
Mexican	Pinto or black beans; fajitas (you decide what goes in them); side salad instead of rice	Fried tortilla chips; beef or cheese burritos; sour cream; fried taco shells; Spanish rice; refried beans
Thai	Broth-based soups; stir-fried, grilled, or steamed dishes; baked or steamed tofu and vegetables	Thai iced tea; dishes made with coconut milk; fried dishes

PERSONAL GOAL

Date: _____ I will:

☐ Practice stopping eating a few bites earlier than I normally would.

☐ Go for a walk to gather menu information on local restaurants or check out the National Restaurant Association's website at www.restaurant.org and search for "Dining Guides."

☐ Order salad dressing, sour cream, butter, and gravy on the side.

☐ Turn down the "Do you want cheese with that?" offer.

☐ Avoid foods prepared with the words "breaded," "crispy," or "creamy."

☐ Request baked or broiled rather than fried.

☐ Ask for a to-go container for half of my order before it arrives.

☐ Graciously pass on offers of unhealthy food.

☐ Other: _____.

I only had one glass of wine;
I just kept filling it up!

DAY 16

 Every Step You Take

You don't have to enroll in an extreme sport to reap the benefits of physical activity. It's the everyday steps you take that can make a world of difference. Did you know that lack of exercise is a major risk factor for heart disease and stroke? More than 60% of adults in the U.S. do not get enough activity and at least 25% are completely inactive during their leisure time.

Challenge yourself to get more steps every day. Invest in a pedometer (either a small battery-powered device that clips to your waistband and counts steps, or get a smartphone app). A pedometer helps raise your awareness of how many steps you're actually taking and provides motivation to get more activity in your daily plan. Build up to 10,000 steps a day.

Where can I get a pedometer?

You can find pedometers at your local pharmacy or on the Internet. Omron (www.omronhealthcare.com) makes an accurate, easy-to-use pedometer that keeps daily averages for a quick comparison of walking trends. The Yamax Digi-Walker pedometers (www.new-lifestyles.com) are also very good. Check out

The Benefits of Walking

- Adding 2,000 steps a day can prevent weight gain. It can help prevent diabetes, so invite your family and friends to join in.
- Taking 2,000 steps burns about 100 calories.
- Americans as a whole average about 5,600 steps a day and have an obesity rate of 22.8%.
- People in Colorado average about 6,500 steps a day, the highest of any state in the U.S., and have an obesity rate of 16%.
- The Amish average about 16,000 steps a day and have an obesity rate of 9%.

www.fitbit.com or download their free app. Regardless of the brand you select, make sure it has—and that you use—a security strap feature to prevent the pedometer from falling off your clothes.

Do I need to get my walking in all at once?

No. The American Diabetes Association's 2013 Standards of Care recommend that adults with diabetes perform at least 150 minutes per week of moderate-intensity aerobic physical activity, spread over at least 3 days per week, and according to the U.S. Physical Activity Guidelines (2008), this can be achieved in episodes of at least 10-minute increments. If you want to lose weight, the National Institutes of Health recommends you do 60 minutes a day most days of the week, follow a nutritious eating plan, and consume fewer calories than you burn each day.

Is running better than walking?

Not necessarily. Walking briskly can provide the same health benefits as running. Runners tend to have more injuries and can miss more days of activity.

Is it okay to use hand weights while walking?

Just leave the hand weights at home. Hand weights can increase blood pressure, which can be dangerous. It's best to weight train separately from walking.

PERSONAL GOAL

Date: _____ I will:

☐ Buy a pedometer and measure the number of steps I take every day.
☐ Start a program of 10 minutes of brisk walking 3 days a week.
☐ Increase to 30 minutes of walking per day at least 5 days a week.
☐ Walk while doing errands rather than relying on my car.
☐ Check out www.americaonthemove.org to find activities in my community.
☐ Write my daily steps on a calendar or track them on an iPhone app, so I can watch my progress.
☐ Don't give up if I miss a few days.
☐ Other: _____.

Walk a mile in his shoes? No thanks.
I'd rather walk two in mine.

DAY 17

 Under Pressure

We tend to focus only on glucose levels in people with diabetes. But did you know that two out of three people with diabetes have high blood pressure (compared with one out of three people without diabetes)? High blood pressure is the most common cause of cardiovascular disease (CVD), a condition that involves the heart or blood vessels. CVD accounted for one of every three deaths in the U.S. for people with and without diabetes, according to the American Heart Association (2013 Statistical Update). Blood vessels travel everywhere in the body, and if the flow is disrupted through a partial or complete blockage, it can lead to a heart attack or stroke. People with diabetes who also have ongoing high cholesterol and glucose levels are at a higher-than-average risk of having a heart attack or stroke. That's serious business, yet you can minimize your risk with your daily behaviors that help to manage diabetes, blood pressure and cholesterol (stay tuned for more info on cholesterol on Day 22; let's focus on blood pressure for now).

What is blood pressure?

Blood pressure is the measurement of the force of blood as it presses against the walls of your arteries. The medical term for high blood pressure is hypertension. Hypertension puts extra strain on the heart and can damage small blood vessels in the kidneys and eyes. The blood pressure is recorded as two numbers:
- The systolic, or "top number," is the force exerted when your heart is contracting (pumping).
- The diastolic, or "bottom number," is the force present when your heart is at rest (between beats).

The target blood pressure for people with diabetes is less than 140/80 mmHg.

What causes hypertension?

In general, you are more likely to develop hypertension if you—
- Have a family history of hypertension
- Are overweight
- Don't exercise
- Have unrelieved stress
- Eat too much salt
- Drink too much alcohol
- Are African American
- Smoke

You can do several things to help keep your blood pressure healthy:
- Eat wisely. Choose lots of fresh vegetables and fruits, whole-grain breads, cereals, and pasta. Avoid fried foods and those with high fat. Cut down on sodium, caffeine, and alcohol.
- Engage in regular physical activity according to your ability. (Certainly avoid inactivity!)
- Manage stress.
- Stop smoking and stay away from secondhand smoke!
- Take medications (several types are available, refer to Week 11).

Have you heard about morning hypertension?

It's a condition in which average weekly blood pressure levels taken within 2 hours after waking in the morning exceed 140/80 mmHg. This can significantly increase your risk for stroke. One of the best ways to know your risk is to check your blood pressure at home (it's okay if you're not ready for this now, as Week 18 covers it).

PERSONAL GOAL

Date: _____ I will:

☐ Ask my health-care provider to take my blood pressure every time I go in.
☐ Buy a home blood pressure monitoring device and get help in figuring out how to use it.
☐ Have a going-away party for the salt shaker.
☐ Mail my cigarettes back to the manufacturer.
☐ Ask about seeing a heart doctor (cardiologist) if I have high blood pressure.
☐ Find a healthy way to relieve stress.
☐ Other: _____.

You'd have high blood pressure too if you had to constantly think about diabetes.

DAY
18

Metformin

Who takes this drug?

People with type 2 diabetes, those with prediabetes, women with a history of gestational diabetes found to have prediabetes, or women with polycystic ovarian syndrome.

What is metformin?

Metformin is the generic name of a diabetes medication that has been used in Europe since the 1960s and became available in the U.S. a few decades later. It belongs to the biguanide class of medications and is available in pill and liquid forms and in combination pills. It can be taken with other diabetes medications, including insulin. You may have heard the trade name of this drug called Glucophage, but since the patent expired, most people use the generic form, metformin.

How does this drug work?

Metformin works by decreasing the amount of glucose production from the liver. It does not cause weight gain and can help lower triglyceride levels. It also may preserve beta-cells. It is taken with or toward the end of a meal. Noticeable changes in blood glucose levels may not be seen until after 2 weeks of consistently taking the drug.

Possible side effects

Bloating, gas, nausea, and diarrhea (usually subside after the first week).

Warning

If you have a liver problem (such as hepatitis), or drink excessive amounts of alcohol, metformin is *not* for you. Metformin may be used in people with stable congestive heart failure (CHF) if the kidney function is normal. It should be avoided in unstable or hospitalized patients with CHF. It should be used cautiously with people more than 80 years old or for those with kidney (renal) insufficiency (as measured in a test called the estimated glomerular filtration rate, or eGFR).

- If the eGFR level is less than 30 (reported as milliliters per minute per 1.73 meters squared—yes, complicated, but you at least get a sense of what the values mean), usually the dose is lowered to half of the maximum, and renal function is monitored every 3 months or the metformin is stopped.
- If the eGFR is more than 30 and less than 45, metformin may be prescribed with caution and renal function monitoring occurs every 3 to 6 months.
- If the eGFR is more than 45 and less than 60, metformin may be continued with yearly renal function test.
- If the eGFR is 60 or more, there are no renal contraindications to metformin.

Your doctor will probably request lab tests to check kidney and liver function before starting you on metformin and monitor these at least annually. A rare, but often fatal, condition called lactic acidosis can occur in certain high-risk groups.

PERSONAL GOAL

Date: _____ I will:

☐ Take my metformin with food.
☐ Call my provider to report diarrhea, gas, nausea, or bloating that does not go away.
☐ Continue to take metformin if my glucose is in target range, unless my doctor advises otherwise.
☐ Tell my health-care provider if I stop taking my medication, regardless of the reason.
☐ Plan for what to do when I forget my dose. Take my metformin if it is within 3 hours of the scheduled dose (with a snack). Otherwise, I'll skip that dose and take it at the next prescribed time. I won't double up on doses.
☐ Limit alcohol when on metformin (check with my doctor to see if it's okay to have an occasional drink, but stay hydrated when enjoying a little alcohol).
☐ Other: _____.

 I love what you do for me, metformin!

DAY
19

 Check Your Eyes Yearly to See Clearly

How is your vision? Some individuals newly diagnosed with diabetes report a worsening of eyesight or blurriness. After glucose levels return to an ideal range, vision tends to improve yet you need to know how to keep your eyes protected. The only way to know if your eyes are safe is to have a comprehensive and dilated eye exam by an ophthalmologist or optometrist. This is recommended shortly after the diabetes diagnosis and every 2–3 years following a normal eye exam (more frequently for any signs of retinopathy, a topic covered in Week 46).

What's the difference between an optometrist and an ophthalmologist?

An ophthalmologist is a physician who specializes in the medical and surgical care of the eyes and visual system. An optometrist is a doctor of optometry who examines, diagnoses, and manages diseases of the eye and visual system. Both of these specialists can examine your eyes, but only an ophthalmologist can perform surgery. Optometrists can check your eyesight and help with minor eye problems. Opticians specialize in eyewear. You may see all three in the course of taking care of your eyes.

What signs should I watch for?

Often, there are no early signs of vision problems. Report any of the following problems to your doctor:
- Blurred or double vision
- Pain or pressure in the eyes
- Flashing lights or rings of light in the vision
- Difficulty seeing things out of the corner of the eyes

How can my doctor check my visual ability?

Three main types of examinations are used to determine eye health.

1. *Visual acuity test.* That eye chart that you read from a distance with different rows of letters and numbers; it checks if you have 20/20 vision.
2. *Dilated eye exam.* Eyedrops are used to widen your pupils so that the doctor can check your retina and optic nerve for damage by using a special magnifying lens.
3. *Tonometry.* This test measures eye pressure and can indicate whether you have glaucoma or other pressure-related problems.

PERSONAL GOAL

Date: _____ I will:

☐ Call my ophthalmologist or optometrist to make an appointment for my dilated eye exam (or find one by calling Eye Care America at 877-887-6327).

☐ Check my blood glucose if my vision suddenly becomes blurry.

☐ Give up smoking or secondhand smoke to keep the tiny blood vessels in my eyes healthy.

☐ Give some thought to what my doctor said about starting that blood pressure pill!

☐ Reduce my fat intake, which will lower my cholesterol and help me keep my eyes healthy.

☐ Keep my eyes lubricated—if they are dry—with a normal saline-type solution (not brands that advertise reducing redness).

☐ If I'm planning on pregnancy, I'll have an eye exam in my first trimester with close follow-up throughout my pregnancy and for 1 year after giving birth.

☐ Other: _____.

 I can see clearly now, the cake is gone.

DAY
20

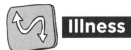 **Illness**

What does getting sick have to do with this?

It is a wild card (and not a good one!) that can send you to the hospital, but not if you know what to do. This topic is presented early on to keep you safe.

Your glucose can go up and it has nothing to do with food

Food is the not the only reason blood glucose levels rise. Under periods of stress, our fight-or-flight hormones (such as adrenaline) give our bodies extra energy to defend ourselves (or run away). Extra glucose pours in from the liver to fight off attackers, regardless of whether that attacker is a bear, a bacteria or virus, emotions, or that thing causing stress (including pain).

Your glucose can stabilize only to be sent into a tailspin when you catch a cold. When you don't feel well, it is hard to stay on top of your diabetes plan, but this can mean the difference between staying at home with instructions on what to do, versus a visit to the physician's office or a trip to the hospital.

At what point should I be worried and call the doctor?

If you have a persistent fever, nausea or vomiting, diarrhea that lasts more than 6 hours, blood glucose levels less than 70 mg/dL on any given day that you are sick, or blood glucose levels more than 250 mg/dL for two consecutive days. Granted, you were recently diagnosed, so your blood glucose levels already may be in the 200 mg/dL range, so ask your health-care provider when you should call.

What if I am too sick to eat?

Your body still needs energy during periods of illness. You may not be able to follow your meal plan if you are feeling nauseated. In situations like this, try eating foods high in carbohydrate and monitoring blood glucose levels more frequently. That way, you'll still get some energy from your meals, even if they're tiny. Examples of foods to choose when you are sick include the following:

- 1 cup of soup or noodles
- 1/2 cup of regular soda
- 1/2 cup of juice
- 6 saltine crackers
- 1/2 cup of ice cream, sherbet, or sorbet (or popsicles!)

Try to stay hydrated because dehydration can make your blood glucose levels go crazy. Drink calorie-free liquids, such as water, tea, and broth.

Have a sick-day plan

The best way to avoid problems when you're sick is to have a plan. Stock up with some key items, so you will be prepared for most situations. Have sugar-free cough drops and fever medicine available. Have a list of contact information for your health-care providers handy so you can call if you have questions. You'll also need to have a plan for handling your medications when ill. You may need to change your dosages. Discuss these issues with your health-care team beforehand, and you will avoid many unpleasant surprises.

PERSONAL GOAL

Date: _____ I will:

☐ Get supplies I will need when I'm sick, such as sugar-free cough drops, fever medicine, over-the-counter pain medicine (that has been approved by my physician), soup, saltine crackers, small boxes of juice, tea, and other beverages.

☐ Check my blood glucose at least every 4 hours when I don't feel well.

☐ Call my health-care provider when my blood glucose levels are more than 250 mg/dL for more than 2 days or if I have one reading of less than 70 mg/dL.

☐ Ask my health-care provider about flu and other vaccines, and how to handle medications during periods of illness.

☐ Put together a list of important phone numbers, so I am prepared if I need to make an emergency call.

☐ Take a sick day from work if I am ill.

☐ Other: _____.

Why do I have to be sick to enjoy a little guilt-free ice cream?

DAY 21

 From Depression to Refreshin'

You have a whole book in front of you with suggestions on how to make changes in your life with diabetes and you may well be feeling overwhelmed about it! You may have been told you need to lose weight and make changes to your diet and exercise routines, which could make you feel guilty about your current lifestyle. Does having diabetes ever make you feel ashamed, embarrassed, or stressed out? You are not alone and you can feel better with a little help.

It is common for people with diabetes to feel some distress related to the burden of managing diabetes. Sometimes, these feelings of distress go beyond a bad day. How's your mood? What do you do for fun? High levels of distress and depression are two different conditions; both are common with diabetes and merit explanation.

What is depression?

Depression is much more than occasionally feeling blue or being sad. If you've suddenly found that you couldn't care less about the things that you used to love, that's a sign of depression. People with diabetes are twice as likely to have depressive symptoms than people without diabetes.

Depression is a syndrome with nine symptoms, at least five of which need to be present nearly every day for at least 2 weeks. Take a look at the list below and see if any of these apply to you on a regular basis.

One of these:
- Depressed mood
- Loss of interest and pleasure

Plus four of these:
- Change in sleep patterns

- Change in appetite or weight
- Low energy or fatigue
- The body doesn't want to do what the mind tells it to do
- Lack of concentration
- Thoughts of suicide or death

Does any of this sound familiar? If so, seek help from your health-care team.

I don't need to see a psychotherapist

People often groan at the mention of psychotherapy, but consider this: A scientific study showed that 85% of people with depression and diabetes reported no more episodes of depression after weekly hour-long sessions of cognitive behavioral therapy with a psychotherapist for 10 weeks. Although psychotherapy is often socially stigmatized, it is an effective way to treat depression.

Benefits of Treating Depression

- No more depression
- Improved sleep and eating patterns
- Reduced pain
- Increased social and physical activity
- Better coping ability
- Improved blood glucose control

Could you have diabetes distress?

As described by Dr. Larry Fisher, diabetes can be tough and cause a range of hassles from minor to major life difficulties. During the past month, how bothersome were the following? Use a scale from not a problem at all, to a slight, moderate, serious or very serious problem.

1. Feeling overwhelmed by the demands of living with diabetes?
2. Feeling that I am often failing with my diabetes routine?

It is normal to feel burdened from time to time with this disease, especially with all the annoying details just provided to you over the past few weeks! Factors that contribute to this are related to the emotional toll, treatment plan (and how complex it is), physician-related distress, and interpersonal distress. This is important to know so that you can recognize when it is happening to you, then you can decide whether and when to reach out to your personal network for support.

PERSONAL GOAL

Date: _____ I will:

- ☐ Remind myself that it is not my fault that I have diabetes, and that managing it is a hard job—one I never even applied for.
- ☐ Ask a friend or loved one to join me in a walk and talk about what feelings come up for me around my diabetes.
- ☐ Do for myself what I would normally do for someone else.
- ☐ Next time I see a number that is out of range on my meter, realize it is a number and give myself a break.
- ☐ Strive for consistency, not perfection, with my diabetes self-care.
- ☐ Find a therapist (ask my health-care team and insurance company; contact the National Mental Health Association at 800-969-6642 or www.nmha.org/affiliates/directory/index.cfm; or talk with my school counselor, minister, rabbi, or imam).
- ☐ Check my insurance coverage for mental health care.
- ☐ Call the National Hopeline Network Crisis Center at 800-442-4673 if I need help immediately.
- ☐ Discuss symptoms of depression with my health-care providers.
- ☐ Check out "10 Things You Should Know About Depression" at behavioraldiabetesinstitute.org.

 I'm so bummed I couldn't care less, but I end up caring about being so bummed.

WEEK 3: REVIEW

Date: _____

Some of the changes you've brought into your life to help manage your diabetes will have become good habits.

Flip back through the past 3 weeks of your personal goals and review.

1. Which goal was completed without much thought or effort?
   _____
   _____

2. Which goal did you forget that you had made?_____
   _____

3. In which area did you surprise yourself with your ability to manage? _____
   _____

4. How often are you checking your glucose each day?_____
   _____
   _____

5. Are your glucose numbers improving overall? _____

6. Write down any patterns you see in your glucose results to discuss with your provider (e.g., high readings in the morning, in range before dinner, high at bedtime, low after a walk):_____
   _____

7. Enter my weight: _____

WEEK 4

Laughin' Langerhans

By Theresa Garnero

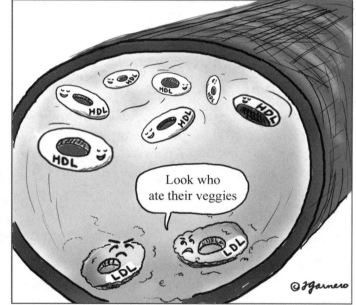

Inside your blood vessels . . .

DAY
22

 Fat Chance

Why focus so much on how I eat?

Even though many people with diabetes find it difficult to adjust eating patterns, one study found that making changes in your diet will have a greater impact on your diabetes control than making changes in your exercise levels. Of course, regular physical activity helps on *so* many levels and is an integrated focus throughout this book. The point is, if you are having difficulty focusing on one area, learning how to eat in ways that are consistently healthy and enjoyable will give you long-lasting benefits.

I've been watching carbohydrates so closely that I haven't paid any attention to cholesterol

Learning about healthy nutrition is like understanding a new language. You build on the basics, try not to incorporate too much at one time to avoid getting overwhelmed, keep practicing, and then one day you find yourself speaking that new language. Cholesterol is an important basic concept to grasp.

What is cholesterol?

Cholesterol is a waxy substance made by the liver that moves through your bloodstream and helps your cells function. Your body usually makes all of the cholesterol it needs, but your food choices add extra cholesterol to the bloodstream and contribute to plaque buildup within the arteries. Let's turn our focus to improving the quality of the fat you consume.

Fats, fats, and more fats!

Remember that *all* fats have *twice* the number of calories as carbohydrates or protein. There are several different kinds, some to enjoy without guilt, others to limit or avoid.

What are omega-3 and omega-6 fats?

The omega fats are called essential fatty acids because you can only get them from your diet. Studies show that to stay healthy, you should consume more omega-3 fats than omega-6 fats. You need both types.

Most omega-3 fats help reduce inflammation in major body systems (like the cardiovascular, circulatory, neurological, and gastrointestinal systems). Omega-3 fats are found in fish (particularly fatty fish like salmon, mackerel, herring, lake trout, sardines, and albacore tuna). Other excellent sources are walnuts, flax seeds, and pumpkin seeds.

Omega-6 fatty acids help promote inflammation in the body. Healthy sources of omega-6 are whole-grain breads, poultry, eggs, cereal, nuts, seeds, and some vegetable and seed oils. Unhealthy sources loaded with omega-6 are cookies, candy, cake, fast food, fried food, crackers, and chips.

Consuming more omega-6 than omega-3 puts the body at

Healthier Fats (can lower blood cholesterol)*

Monounsaturated fats are found in olive, canola, and peanut oil; avocados; seeds; and most nuts, such as almonds, peanuts, cashews, and hazelnuts.

Polyunsaturated fats are found in sunflower, safflower, corn, soybean, sesame, flaxseed, and cottonseed oils; some fish (such as salmon, mackerel, albacore tuna, sardines, and trout); and walnuts.

*When substituted for unhealthy fats.

Avoidable Fats (can raise blood cholesterol)

Saturated fats are found in animal products (including dairy, chicken, meat) and tropical oils (coconut, cocoa butter, and palm). They are usually solid at room temperature. Do your best to decrease the amount of saturated fat in your diet.

Trans fats or hydrogenated fats are found in most baked goods, cookies, pastries, pies, fast foods, shortening, and stick margarine. They also lurk in most processed foods (look for "hydrogenated fats" on the label). Trans fats are sometimes called trans fatty acids.

increased risk for conditions like heart disease, cancer, high blood pressure, diabetes, and arthritis. What does this mean? Eat more omega-3 than omega-6 by eating more fresh foods and veggies like broccoli, cauliflower, kale, cabbage, Brussels sprouts, and nonfat milk, and by reducing your consumption of processed and fast foods and polyunsaturated vegetable oils (corn, sunflower, safflower, soy, and cottonseed).

Smart choices for healthy cholesterol

CHOOSE OFTEN*			
Helps improve your cholesterol levels			
Olives	Peanut oil	Broccoli	Salmon
Olive oil	Avocados	Zucchini	Mackerel
Seeds: pumpkin and sunflower	Nuts (almonds, peanuts)	Chard	Sardines
Canola oil	Spinach	Oils (sunflower, soybean, cottonseed)	Tuna

*In a low-fat diet. Too much of any fat can increase your cholesterol.

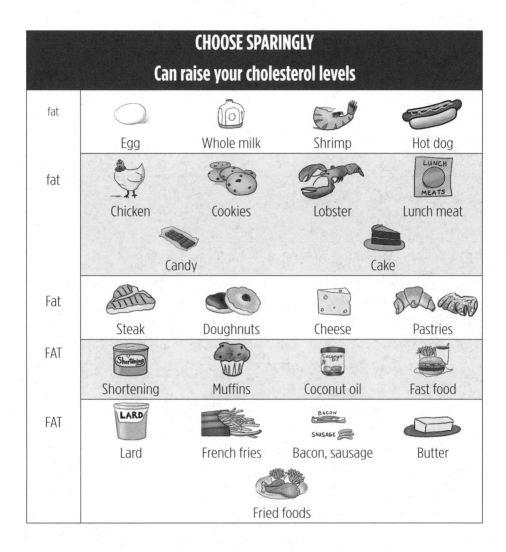

CHOOSE SPARINGLY
Can raise your cholesterol levels

fat	Egg	Whole milk	Shrimp	Hot dog
fat	Chicken	Cookies	Lobster	Lunch meat
	Candy		Cake	
Fat	Steak	Doughnuts	Cheese	Pastries
FAT	Shortening	Muffins	Coconut oil	Fast food
FAT	Lard	French fries	Bacon, sausage	Butter
		Fried foods		

What's better: butter or margarine?

Check out this chart and decide which is better.

Comparison of Butter and Margarines (1 tablespoon)

	Butter	Stick margarine	Tub margarine	Smart Balance	Benecol
Calories	110	100	60	80	70
Fat	12 grams	11 grams	7 grams	9 grams	8 grams
Saturated Fat	8 grams	2.5 grams	1.5 grams	2.5 grams	1 gram
Trans Fat	0	3 grams	0	0	0
Cholesterol	30 mg	0	0	0	0

Source: *The Diabetes Carbohydrate & Fat Gram Guide*, by Lea Ann Holzmeister, RD, CDE.

Have you heard of plant sterols?

Plant sterols are components of cell membranes in many fruits, legumes, nuts, seeds, and vegetables. Many recent studies have shown that plant sterols can lower your cholesterol levels. It can be a challenge to add plant sterols to your diet, but you can find it in some fortified foods and beverages.

PERSONAL GOAL

Date: _____ I will:

☐ Double the amount of fresh vegetables in my diet.
☐ Use low-fat (1% or 2%) or fat-free milk.
☐ Remove the skin from poultry and trim any fat from meats.
☐ Try a vegetarian dish.
☐ Bake, steam, roast, grill, or broil dishes instead of frying them.
☐ Use lemon or herb seasonings to flavor dishes instead of butter or margarine.
☐ Eat less cheese or switch to reduced-fat or light cheese.
☐ Skip bacon, sausage, and fast food for a week.
☐ Ask for the salad dressing on the side.
☐ Cut down on pastries, cakes, cookies, and junk food.
☐ Appreciate that milk (even lactose-free) has carbs.
☐ Limit egg yolks to three per week.
☐ Other:_____.

 These pants no longer fit my trans fanny.

Cholesterol Quotas

My doctor watches my cholesterol, so my numbers must be okay.

Are you sure? Elevated levels of cholesterol (also known as hyperlipidemia) and high blood pressure are a double threat to your heart. Knowing your numbers is the first step toward maintaining your health. Typically, high cholesterol has no symptoms. The American Diabetes Association recommends an annual lipid panel (a simple blood test) taken to check your cholesterol.

Okay, so what's total cholesterol?

Total cholesterol represents the total amount of cholesterol circulating in your blood at the time of the test. It includes HDL and LDL (described in the following sections). In general, you want your total cholesterol to be less than 200 mg/dL, but it doesn't give you the detail you need. Focus on HDL and LDL in the following sections.

HDL cholesterol stands for *healthy*

The HDL stands for "high-density lipoprotein." HDL cholesterol is known as the "healthy" or "good" cholesterol because it lowers the levels of "bad" or "lousy" cholesterol. Ideal levels are more than 40 mg/dL for men and more than 50 mg/dL for women. You can raise your HDL cholesterol level by being active on a regular basis, controlling your weight, and quitting smoking.

LDL cholesterol stands for *lousy*

LDL stands for "low-density lipoprotein" and is known as the "lousy" or "bad" cholesterol because it clogs up the walls of your arteries with small, sticky particles of cholesterol. This often is called plaque and can lead to strokes and heart attacks. Ideal levels for LDL cholesterol are less than 100 mg/dL (less than 70 mg/dL if you already have cardiovascular disease). If you are on maximal tolerated statin therapy (you'll learn more about statins in Week 16), an alternative therapeutic LDL goal is 30–40% lower than your initial baseline. Lower your LDL by eating foods with less saturated fat, trans fat, and cholesterol and by taking medication, if needed.

What are triglycerides?

Triglycerides are considered free fatty acids, which can be very useful in the body at appropriate levels, but they are harmful if levels rise more than 150 mg/dL. You may see "triglycerides" shortened to TG on lab reports, which are also the author's initials. Consider it my way of sending you love on your lab report! The ideal level for triglycerides is less than 150 mg/dL. You can lower your triglyceride level by exercising, eating less sugar and white starches or grains, drinking less alcohol (if you drink more than moderately), and keeping your blood glucose under control. Medication may be needed.

What's this new test, Apo B?

Studied for the past few decades and now available in mainstream use, Apolipoprotein B (Apo B) is another blood test that measures the very tiny, dense proteins attached to LDL cholesterol; both travel through the bloodstream. These small Apo B molecules can clog arteries even more so than LDL because they are very small and can get into places that LDL cannot. Apo B levels are used, along with other lipid tests, to help determine one's risk of developing CVD. It provides a better measure of cardiac risk than does LDL alone.

When is it ordered?

Apo B levels are checked when someone has a family history of heart disease or has very high triglyceride levels (which can prevent the accurate calculation of LDL levels). Apo B levels are also useful in monitoring the effect of cholesterol-lowering medications, called statins (covered in Week 16), which lower LDL and these harmful Apo B molecules.

How often do I need to have my cholesterol checked?

For adults, check fasting lipid levels at least once a year. Some health-care providers monitor lipid levels four times a year until goals are reached.

PERSONAL GOAL

Date: _____ I will:

☐ Get copies of my most recent cholesterol readings and write in my results below.
   Date of test: _____
   Total cholesterol level _____ mg/dL
   HDL cholesterol level _____ mg/dL
   LDL cholesterol level _____ mg/dL
   Triglyceride level _____ mg/dL
   Apo B level _____ mg/dL

☐ Ask my health-care provider about having a lipid panel taken.

☐ If I don't have insurance or access to health care, contact my hospital or pharmacy to see when they have free cholesterol screenings or get a BioSafe Cholesterol Panel Test at the pharmacy, so I can take a cholesterol test at home.

☐ I will cut back on drinking alcohol to no more than one drink for women or two drinks for men daily.

☐ Quit smoking or get away from secondhand smoke.

☐ Get 30 minutes of physical activity today.

☐ Other:_____.

How fat is your blood?

DAY
24

 And...Action!

Americans stare at a screen on average for 8 hours a day, more time than we spend on any other activity including sleeping, according to the *Newsweek* article, "Tweet. Texts. Email. Posts. Is the Onslaught Making Us Crazy?" About 50% of our population's increase in weight has been associated with too much screen time (television and computer or tablet viewing). Each hour spent staring at a screen increases the risk of being overweight. Cutting that time to fewer than 10 hours per week and increasing physical activity to 30 minutes a day can help prevent diabetes and prevent obesity. Tell that to our kids and then try to practice what we preach. Check out these astounding stats:

- **Children:** Approximately 30% ages 2–6 years have a television in their room. This keeps kids away from healthier activities, such as family time, playing outside, and getting sleep. Children as young as 2 years old see more than 20,000 television commercials a year, often promoting foods and beverages that are high in fats, sugar, or salt. The average U.S. child spends about 1,000 more hours per year in front of a screen than in school.
- **Teens:** average 3,700 texts a month and 7 hours of screen time into a typical school day.
- **Adults:** average 8 hours of screen time per day; by the time the average American reaches age 65 years, *an entire 9 years* will have been spent watching television.

Where you are now, versus where we all should be

Looking at the scale of "not being active at all" to "active for 30 minutes a day," how do you rate?

Physical activity standards in a perfect world?

The standard is 150 minutes a week, which includes the following:

- At least 3 days a week, moderate-intensity aerobic activity (50–70% of maximum heart rate), with no more than 2 consecutive days without exercise.
- Muscle-strengthening activities that involve all major muscle groups at least twice per week and not on consecutive days. These resistance-training sessions with free weights, weight machines, or elastic bands consist of at least one set of five or more different resistance exercises involving the larger muscle groups.

What's the best exercise?

Motivated? The best exercise is the one that you're most likely to enjoy doing on a regular basis. The ultimate goal is to not go more than 2 consecutive days without exercise. When choosing an exercise, think about your goals (weight loss, good health, participate in a team sport, or training for a competition), your interests, and your schedule. The ideal exercise program will include aerobic, resistance (strength), and flexibility. Let's review:

Aerobic. Periods of continuous, aerobic (oxygen-requiring) exercise, preferably for at least 30 minutes three or more times a week. And it doesn't have to be one, 30-minute activity! You can also accomplish this by shorter, 10-minute bouts of activity. Examples include those that use large muscle groups: brisk walking, jumping rope, cycling, rowing, swimming, cross-country skiing, figure skating, rollerblading, and jogging.

Resistance training. Also known as strength training, these are repeated contractions or forced exertion of major muscle groups for a brief amount of time, preferably at least twice a week. Examples include weight lifting, resistance bands, push-ups, and sit-ups. Unless you have been advised not to, do 10 repetitions, also referred to as one "set," and three sets per type of exercise.

Flexibility. This is your muscles' and joints' ability to move through a full range of motion. For example, sitting and reaching toward your toes measures the flexibility of your lower back and hamstrings (the back part of your upper legs). Best done after a brief warm-up and in combination with aerobic and resistance training exercises. Stretch only to the point of tightness (not pain) at least 15 seconds per stretch and include upper- and lower-body muscle groups.

Benefits of exercise include the following:

Increases energy level and your ability to control your weight

Decreases glucose, blood pressure, cholesterol, stress, and depression

Makes your insulin work **better** and may reduce your need for diabetes medication

Decreases your risk for heart problems and stroke (the leading causes of complications for people with *uncontrolled* diabetes)

PERSONAL GOAL

Date: _____ I will:

☐ Get up and stretch at least every hour while in front of a screen.

☐ Cut out 30 minutes of television time a day.

☐ Write down how much television I watch and how many steps I take every day.

☐ Stop eating in front of the television.

☐ Avoid watching any television for an entire day.

☐ Take a Facebook vacation for a week.

Other: _____.

Can I help it if I like watching cooking shows and triathlons?

DAY
25

Insulin Secretagogues

Who takes this drug?

Insulin secretagogues are used by people with type 2 diabetes.

What is an insulin secretagogue?

A group of medications that cause the pancreas to release more insulin. Several different types are available, including combination pills.

- Amaryl (glimepiride)
- Micronase, Diabeta, or Glynase (glyburide)
- Glucotrol (glipizide)
- Prandin (repaglinide)
- Starlix (nateglinide)

How do insulin secretagogues work?

These drugs knock on the front door of the pancreas and demand that insulin come out and go into the bloodstream. They often are used in combination with other medications that lower glucose, such as biguanides (Glucophage), thiazolidinediones (such as Actos), and long-acting insulin (such as Lantus or Levemir). If the pancreas does not have enough insulin-producing beta-cells, insulin segretagogues don't help.

Possible side effects

Hypoglycemia (blood glucose less than 70 mg/dL) with symptoms (such as irritability, shakiness, sweating, dizziness, fast heartbeat, hunger, blurred vision, weakness, drowsiness, or difficulty walking or talking).

Warning

These drugs can cause prolonged hypoglycemia (up to 72 hours) in the elderly or in those with kidney problems. Some may experience slight weight gain. The increased risk of hypoglycemia makes it important to take them with food. Alcohol also should be avoided. If you take an insulin secretagogue, be prepared to treat hypoglycemia with a rapidly absorbed carbohydrate source, such as fast-acting glucose.

PERSONAL GOAL

Date: _____ I will:

☐ Carry 15 grams of a rapidly absorbed carbohydrate source such as fast-acting glucose with me at all times (four glucose tablets, a small box of raisins, a small juice box, or a small tube of frosting). Have other sources at home such as a tablespoon of honey, or a 0.68-ounce tube of icing decorating gel (but you'll need a scissors to cut the top of the tube).

☐ Limit alcohol if I am taking an insulin secretagogue.

☐ Report unexplained lows to my doctor.

☐ Ask my health-care provider to suggest another medication if my blood glucose levels are still high on these drugs.

☐ Other:_____.

 Insulin secretagogues are not places of worship.

DAY 26

 Go Nuts! Or Have a Snack

The rich and delicious flavor of nuts can be used to substitute or replace meat and beans in your diet, and can be an excellent source of unsaturated fats and protein. When buying nuts, select ones that are fresh, dry roasted, and unsalted. Store nuts in an airtight container (they can last up to 6 months in the refrigerator and up to 1 year in the freezer). They also can be a helpful snack.

Snack Ideas

Small snacks can keep you going in between meals and help you eat mindfully. Some ideas to consider, courtesy of Kathy Solis, RD, MS, CDE, include the following:

Pears and Cheese

Carb: 1/2 large pear
Protein: 1 ounce light brie cheese

NUTRITION INFORMATION
130 calories, 4.5 grams total fat (2.5 grams saturated fat), 15 milligrams cholesterol, 230 milligrams sodium, 15 grams carb, 3 grams fiber, 7 grams protein

Raisins and Seeds

Carb: 1 mini box raisins
Protein: 2 tablespoons dry-roasted pumpkin seeds

NUTRITION INFORMATION
145 calories, 8 grams total fat (1.5 grams saturated fat), 0 milligrams cholesterol, 50 milligrams sodium, 14 grams carb, 3.5 grams fiber, 5 grams protein

Quick-and-Easy Quesadilla

Carb: 2 thin yellow corn tortillas
Protein: 1/4 cup finely shredded reduced-fat cheddar cheese
Microwave to melt the cheese. Serve with 1/4 cup low-sodium salsa, which counts as a free food (under 20 calories, and less than 5 grams of carbohydrate).

NUTRITION INFORMATION
160 calories, 7 grams total fat (3.5 grams saturated fat), 20 milligrams cholesterol, 200 milligrams sodium, 16 grams carb, 2 grams fiber, 9 grams protein

Open-Face Bagel Melt

Carb: 1/2 thin whole-wheat bagel, toasted
Protein: 1 slice reduced-fat Swiss cheese + 1 slice roasted turkey breast

NUTRITION INFORMATION
145 calories, 5.5 grams total fat (2.5 grams saturated fat), 23 milligrams cholesterol, 267 milligrams sodium, 12 grams carb, 2.5 grams fiber, 13 grams protein

Aim for snacks with about the following:
- 15 grams of carb
- 100–200 calories
- less than 100 milligrams of sodium ideal (max 250 milligrams)
- 5–8 grams of fat

PERSONAL GOAL

Date: _____ I will:

☐ Spread hummus on warm pita bread.
☐ Toss some chickpeas, kidney beans, and pecans on a green salad instead of meat or cheese.
☐ Add toasted almonds, peanuts, or cashews to a veggie stir-fry instead of meat.
☐ Increase vitamin E intake by choosing sunflower seeds, almonds, or hazelnuts.
☐ Lean toward the lean (with round steaks, round roasts, top loin, top sirloin, tenderloin, pork loin, ham, at least 90% lean ground beef, and skinless chicken breast).
☐ Avoid "self-basting" products (chicken, turkey, and pork products that are packed in salt).
☐ Limit liver and other organ meats, as they are high in cholesterol.
☐ Other:_____.

 Butter is a discretionary calorie.
I never was discreet.

DAY 27

 Kidney Kindness

Wouldn't I know if something was wrong with my kidneys?

Early kidney disease typically has no symptoms. Late stages of kidney disease can be accompanied by swelling, weight gain due to fluid retention, poor appetite, fatigue, headache, itchiness, and very little urine output. The longer you have diabetes, the higher your risk for kidney problems, and hence the need to focus on prevention.

Lean, mean, filtering machines

Your kidneys are like super vacuum cleaners that remove toxins and waste from the blood. Each kidney has more than a million tiny blood vessels called nephrons that continuously filter blood. All of the blood in your body passes through the kidneys about 20 times every hour. The kidneys remove water and waste and get rid of it by producing urine. They also return the water that has been filtrated back into the bloodstream, thus maintaining the body's water balance.

What are my chances of having kidney problems?

Recent studies suggest that approximately 20% of people with diabetes develop kidney disease (also called nephropathy). Although all people with diabetes are at risk, some factors are associated with an increased risk of developing nephropathy:

- Certain ethnicities, especially African Americans, Asian Americans, Mexican Americans, and Native Americans
- Smoking
- Long-term high blood glucose levels
- High blood pressure

You can't change your family, but you can do things to change your blood glucose, blood pressure, and exposure to smoke.

Get your urine albumin and blood creatinine checked!

Following are two simple tests that screen for early signs of kidney changes:

1. Urine albumin: a urine test measuring the amount of protein (called albumin). This is done upon diagnosis and annually thereafter.
2. Creatinine: a blood test that also is recommended annually. The creatinine level is used to determine the eGFR, which helps to understand what level, if any, of chronic kidney disease is present.

Kidney care

How you can protect your kidneys:

- Keep blood glucose in the target range as much as possible (even though "diabetes control" is somewhat of an oxymoron, do your best).
- Control blood pressure to less than 140/80 mmHg (cut down on salt to help).
- Avoid exposure to smoke!
- Stay hydrated, if your doctor says your kidneys can handle it. Drinking plenty of water helps your kidneys function properly, just like changing the oil in your car helps it run efficiently.
- Have blood tests performed to check the overall function of your kidneys, including the blood tests called blood urea nitrogen (BUN).
- Exercise regularly (don't let 2 days pass without moving your beautiful body).
- Maintain a healthy weight (or chip away at it every day).
- Discuss other medications you are taking with your physician or pharmacist.
- If you have kidney disease, ask a dietitian for guidance on food choices, and if needed, on a reduction in protein and fluid restriction.

When bad things happen to good kidneys, the goal is to minimize further damage. Hypoglycemia can occur if the kidneys begin to lose their ability to filter out insulin. Other signs of worsening kidney disease include escalating blood pressure, increased potassium levels (hyperkalemia), and anemia (low blood count).

Imagine what your home would look like if you couldn't take out the garbage ever again. For kidneys that have failed, dialysis is like an arrangement to have the trash removed by other people. No one wants dialysis. That would be like wanting a root canal, but it's a vital and necessary procedure when kidneys need help.

PERSONAL GOAL

Date: _____ I will:

☐ Ask to have my kidney tests done (urine albumin; blood creatinine, eGFR, and BUN tests) and get copies of the results.
☐ Report any problems with my urine right away (pain, burning, urgency, frequency, difficulty, blood or pus in the urine).
☐ Avoid exposure to smoke (quit or get away from smokers).
☐ Fill up my large water bottle and drink it every day.
☐ Ask my doctor if I need to restrict my protein intake (see a dietitian for a specialized plan).
☐ Bring all of my medications to my pharmacist to ask if any are tough on my kidneys.
☐ Other: _____.

 Don't kid around with my kidneys.

DAY 28

You've Got Mail...and Strips

Did you know that you can get your diabetes care supplies by mail order? It's a convenient option that may save you time and money. Many companies offer to bill your insurance, pay for shipping, handle all of the paperwork, ensure that your strips and medications don't run out, and provide educational material at no charge. Some are full-service pharmacies that allow you to obtain your medications and products up front without having to pay out of pocket and wait for insurance reimbursement. (If you are ordering insulin by mail, though, be aware of the conditions it may face during shipping—the heat in hot summer months or freezing temperatures in the winter can damage the insulin.)

PERSONAL GOAL

Date: _____ I will:

☐ See whether my health insurance or local pharmacy offers a mail order service (and if they bill insurance).

☐ Ask my health-care provider for a prescription for all diabetes medication and supplies to send to my mail-order company.

☐ Other:_____.

I loved my talking meter until it told me to take out the trash.

DAY
29

Floss to Your Future

Isn't dental care important for everyone? What's different for people with diabetes?

People with diabetes have twice the risk of developing gum disease and teeth problems than the general public. There is a direct link between gum disease and increased mortality rates from cardiovascular and kidney disease. Keep your teeth and gums clean and you will help keep your heart and kidneys happy.

Moreover, people with diabetes who receive treatment for gum disease can enjoy substantial reductions in hospitalizations, doctor visits, and annual medical expenses, according to a study conducted by the University of Pennsylvania. The study's results showed that people with type 2 diabetes who received periodontal care had a 33% annual reduction in hospitalizations, made 13% fewer physician visits, and achieved a decrease in their overall annual medical costs by $1,814!

Controlling blood glucose levels and proper dental hygiene are the best ways to prevent tooth and gum problems. When your blood glucose levels are consistently high, your gums become an ideal location for bacteria to collect. If this leads to an infection, your blood glucose levels may go even higher, reducing your ability to heal. If bacteria hang out in the gum margin, you may develop gingivitis, a

Signs and Symptoms of Periodontal Disease

- Red, swollen, tender, or bleeding gums.
- Gums that have receded from the teeth.
- Ongoing bad breath.
- Loose teeth.
- Pus comes out when the gums are pressed.
- Changes in how the teeth fit together.
- Usually not painful for the person with diabetes.

condition that causes the gums to be inflamed and bleed. Left to fester, this can lead to periodontal disease, a chronic inflammatory disease that destroys the gums and bones and can lead to tooth loss. This doesn't happen overnight, so start taking care of those choppers. You may benefit from antiplaque–anti-gingivitis toothpaste or antiseptic mouthwash.

What if I have dentures?

Even with full dentures, it is important to brush your gums, your tongue, and the roof of your mouth every morning before putting in your dentures. To help keep your gums clean, rinse out your mouth with lukewarm saltwater. Check with your dentist about the proper brush and cleaning solution for your dentures as regular toothpaste can scratch dentures. Also, let your dentist know if your dentures aren't fitting well.

PERSONAL GOAL

Date: _____ I will:

☐ Call the dentist for a checkup.
☐ Tell my dentist I have diabetes.
☐ Try an antiplaque–anti-gingivitis toothpaste.
☐ Get a new, soft-bristle toothbrush.
☐ Buy an electric toothbrush.
☐ Brush my teeth for at least 2 minutes and at least twice a day.
☐ Floss my teeth daily. Make sure the string hugs my tooth
   (go up in between the teeth, then over alongside the tooth
   and back down).
☐ Brush my tongue after I brush my teeth.
☐ Other: _____.

 Reading this chapter in February is not an excuse to avoid the dentist!

DAY 30

 Humor Yourself

Diabetes is no laughing matter, yet therapeutic humor can help people manage their diabetes. According to cartoonist Haidee Merritt, who also has type 1 diabetes, "Humor keeps reality at a safe distance."

Some studies have shown that 30 minutes of laughing a day can lower after-meal blood glucose levels, improve the "good" HDL cholesterol levels by 26%, and reduce the harmful C Reactive Proteins, a blood test to indicate levels of inflammation and cardiovascular risk, by 66%.

The stigma of diabetes is often portrayed negatively, and attention focuses only on the seriousness of the disease. You may not think that humor can be a great defense against diabetes, but it may help you maintain your wits and abilities to endure, and thus, ability to manage this for a lifetime.

Humor is vital to health. You don't have to laugh *at* something to reap the benefits of a good, healthy chuckle. You just have to laugh. There are about 1,000 worldwide laugh clubs that meet to laugh. As strange as this may sound, it feels great afterward.

Humor . . .

- Increases endorphins and lowers anxiety.
- Reduces stress, burnout, and pain.
- Improves learning. Those "ha, ha" moments turn into "aha" moments.
- May improve immune function and blood pressure.
- Is used as a weight-loss therapy (11 hours of laughing = 1 pound weight loss).
- Allows for the expression of anger. Language was invented because we need to communicate. Humor was invented as a way to complain. Listen to any comedian: They are complaining! Dealing with a chronic disease can trigger anger, and humor is a wonderful way to process those emotions.
- Is a low-carb source of energy.

Finding Your Funny Bone

1. Be on the lookout for humor—it's everywhere. We often miss out on humorous situations and funny signs because we're so wrapped up in the seriousness of the moment. Pause to look around yourself, and actively search for humor.
2. Allow yourself to be silly. You have to take risks. But be careful not to do or say anything that might be considered offensive.
3. Learn what amuses you. Did you know cartoons are the most universally accepted form of humor?
4. Learn to laugh at yourself.

By shifting your perspective to the lighter side of the health–disease continuum, you can gain the confidence needed to successfully live and manage your diabetes. Who needs more gloom and doom? Search for humor; it can be therapeutic, whether or not it has to do with your diabetes. Your life is much bigger than a disease. Finding the funny may seem foreign. We get used to doing things a certain way. For example, fold your arms. Go ahead. No one is watching. Now fold them the *other* way.

You rarely hear people exclaim, "I'm so thrilled I have diabetes!" Yet it's not uncommon to hear "Diabetes was the best thing that happened to me—I got my health in order." That is certainly not everyone's perspective. Diabetes does take a lot of work, and humor can help you take it in stride. There is always a choice in how you react to any situation. Sometimes it is hard to see that choice because it is reasonable to react in certain ways. As comedian Yakov Smirnoff said, "We see what we seek. We choose what to focus on." You can choose to change directions in your thinking and focus on the positive.

PERSONAL GOAL

Date: _____ I will:

- ☐ Find at least one funny thing today.
- ☐ Smile at the next person I see.
- ☐ Laugh at myself in the mirror tomorrow morning.
- ☐ Accept the diagnosis, but not the negatively portrayed prognosis of diabetes.
- ☐ Commit to focusing on the positive.
- ☐ Go back to my television and watch something funny.
- ☐ Walk to a comedy club.
- ☐ Look for funny titles or names in the paper.
- ☐ Reach beyond myself and do something goofy and out of character.
- ☐ Other:_____.

 Diabetes means I have
a license to be a finicky eater.

MONTH 1: REVIEW

Date: _____

Let's look back over your first 30 days. Complete the following:

- Before-meal readings average _____ mg/dL

- 2 hours after meal readings average _____ mg/dL
  (Before meal target is 70–130 mg/dL; 2 hours after meals is
  less than 180 mg/dL. It takes time to get there.)

- Last blood pressure reading _____ mmHg
  (Target is less than 140/80 mmHg.)

1. What was your highest glucose?_____Lowest?_____
   Do you know why? _____

2. Favorite meal where your glucose went up less than 50
   points _____

3. What type of exercise did you do this past week?
   _____ For how long? _____

4. Do you feel better equipped to deal with your diabetes diagnosis? Why or why not? _____
   _____

5. Did you take your medication on time?
   Circle one: Nearly always   Sometimes   Almost never

6. Did you take care of your teeth and gums? _____
   _____

7. What was the last thing that caused you to burst out laughing?
   _____

MONTH 2

Laughin' Langerhans

By Theresa Garnero

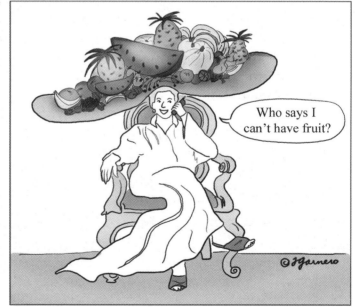

WEEK
5

Carb-o-licious: Milk, Grains, and Desserts

The miracles of milk

In addition to calcium, milk has eight other essential nutrients to keep your body energized. Milk contains vitamin D (which helps the body properly use its calcium and encourages absorption of other essential minerals), riboflavin (a B vitamin that helps convert food into energy), and others, including phosphorus, protein, vitamin B12, potassium, niacin, and vitamin A.

Calcium helps build and maintain healthy bones and prevents osteoporosis, a disease in which the bones become fragile and easily broken. People with diabetes are at a higher risk for osteoporosis. To help keep your bones as strong as they can be, it is essential to have a healthy calcium intake, enough vitamin D3, and regular, yes, exercise. You can ask your health-care provider about checking your vitamin D level. It is often low and can be corrected with careful oversight of vitamin D3 supplementation.

Please know that milk is counted as a carb.

How much milk should I have?

The recommendation is to have two to three servings from the milk group per day. This includes 8 ounces of nonfat or low-fat milk (or plain soymilk or powdered milk) or nonfat yogurt (plain or flavored, with an artificial, non-nutritive sweetener).

What if I don't drink milk? How do I get my calcium?

Vegetable sources of calcium are soybeans, spinach, okra, collard greens, kelp, broccoli, and celery. Other food sources are reduced-fat cheese (1 1/2 to 2 ounces is the equivalent of an 8-ounce glass of milk), calcium-enriched orange juice, and milk substitutes, such as soy, rice, or almond milks. If none of these appeals to you, then taking a calcium and vitamin D3 supplement is an option. Get advice on how much to take. For example, too much calcium can cause kidney stones (ouch!). If you take both calcium and iron supplements, take them at different times.

Pasta, Rice, and Grains—Oh My!

The carbohydrate group also includes grains, cereal, rice, and pasta. Does that mean you can never have white rice, white pasta, or white bread? No, but you are missing out on essential nutrients—like most of the B vitamins and important minerals like magnesium—when you choose refined, white carbohydrates over whole grains. Whenever possible, choose whole-wheat bread (look at the label to be sure this is the first ingredient), whole-wheat flour, brown or wild rice, rolled oats, and whole-grain cereals. (Note: For those allergic to wheat, oats, or rye, advance to Week 31 to learn about gluten-free options, but come back to Week 6!)

Let's talk about grains

A grain is the small, dry, one-seeded fruit of a cereal grass in which the fruit and the seed walls are united. Foods made from wheat, rice, oats, barley, and cornmeal, including bread, cereals, pasta, oatmeal, cereals, tortillas, and grits, are examples of grain products.

- **Whole grains** contain the entire grain kernel (the bran, germ, and endosperm) and include whole-wheat flour, whole-wheat bread or crackers, cracked wheat (bulgur), oatmeal, brown rice, wild rice, whole cornmeal, whole rye, buckwheat, popcorn, and whole-wheat pasta. At least half of your grains should be whole grains.
- **Refined grains** have been processed to remove the bran and germ. Unfortunately, this process also removes a lot of the parts of the grain that are good for you, including the bran, iron, and many B vitamins. Refined grains have a finer texture and longer shelf life and include white flour, white bread, white rice, most pastas, muffins, couscous, flour and corn tortillas, noodles, grits, and pretzels.

How much grain should I eat in a day?

The U.S. Department of Agriculture recommends 14 grams of fiber per 1,000 kcal (translates into about 25–38 grams of fiber per day). Also, at least half of the grains you eat should be whole grains. One way to help you estimate the whole-grain content is to look for the little yellow and black Whole Grain Council stamp on many (but not all) foods. Companies who want to promote the whole grain in their products pay a fee to the Whole Grains Council to let you know how much whole grains are in a product. Each "stamped" product guarantees at least half of a serving (8 grams) of whole grains. Examples of one serving or 16 grams of whole grains include the following: a slice of whole-grain bread; 1/3 cup of cooked whole-wheat pasta (so if you had a cup, you'd get your daily amount); 1/2 of a whole-grain English muffin, 1/3 cup of cooked brown rice, bulgur, or barley; 4 Triscuit crackers; or 2/3 cup of Cheerios. So many numbers! When possible, choose whole grain. Keep in mind grains contain carbs, so check your serving sizes.

Sweet Tooth

Do you have a sweet tooth? Or teeth? Besides the obvious packed-with-a-carb punch, sweets typically include a lot of fat. That's why they taste great, but you know the trouble they can cause when you have diabetes.

What's a net carb?

Some advertising genius thought up the concept of "net carbs" (or "carb impact") because it sells. If you doubt it, just check out the "diabetic food" section at your local grocery store. You think you are getting a low-carb product, but that's not necessarily true. The idea behind net carbs is to subtract the grams of fiber and sugar alcohols from the grams of total carbohydrate to give you the net carbs.

Tackle that Sweet Tooth

- Seek quality, not quantity. If you are craving something in particular, don't compromise. Have a smaller portion and savor it, otherwise you'll end up eating other things without satisfying the beast.
- Make yourself walk to the store to buy treats and don't keep a stash in the house!
- Cut back on other carbs within the meal to make an even trade for the carb in your dessert.
- Out of sight, out of mind. Get help from your spouse or family not to have junk food in the house. (Okay, but it is a strategy!)
- Reduce portion size (skip that gargantuan slice of cake); ask for child-size servings instead or share.
- Have fruit rather than candy.
- Check the calorie and saturated-fat content of your treats.
- Have a glass of water before you start with the dessert (water quenches thirst, not hunger). Doing this makes sure you're not eating when you're actually thirsty.
- Watch out for items labeled "sugar free." By definition, that means the item has less than 1/2 gram of sugar or sucrose in a serving, but it often will contain as many carbohydrates (or more) than the regular product.
- Keep a "sweet" diary and jot down a note of what and how often you are dipping into the proverbial cookie jar.
- Ask yourself whether the reason you are grabbing the sweet is an external solution to stress. That's deep!

PERSONAL GOAL

Date: _____ I will:

☐ Pick milk or water over soda at lunch.
☐ Check the label on bread for carbohydrate and fiber content and to see whether it is whole grain.
☐ Try whole-wheat pasta.
☐ Choose foods that have one of the following whole-grain ingredients listed first on the ingredient list: whole grain, whole wheat, whole oats, whole rye, wild rice, brown rice, graham flour, oatmeal, whole-grain corn, or bulgur.
☐ Try brown or wild rice in place of white rice and cook it up ahead of time to have available as a quick side dish.
☐ Bake some stuffed peppers with a brown rice and mushroom filling.
☐ Add barley to my next soup or stew.
☐ Satisfy my sweet tooth and get calcium with low-fat chocolate milk.
☐ Have popcorn for a snack and instead of salt and butter, sprinkle brewer's yeast.
☐ Other: _____.

 This Halloween, I'm going as a person without diabetes.

WEEK
6

 Glucose Bumps in the Road

Trying to make heads or tails with your blood glucose?

Sometimes there is no rhyme or reason as to what makes glucose go high or low. This week, we'll review some common and not-so-common causes for glucose fluctuations (beyond the reason of "I know I shouldn't have, but I did eat too much Chinese food").

Activity level

If you work your muscles regularly through exercise, you will use insulin more efficiently. As you reduce your insulin resistance, your pancreas won't have to work so hard to make extra insulin (or you won't have to take as much of it) and your glucose levels will adjust in response.

Dawn phenomenon

The dawn phenomenon is the body's response to hormones released in the early morning hours. This occurs for everyone. When we sleep, hormones are released to help maintain and restore cells within our bodies and cause blood glucose levels to rise. For people with diabetes who do not have enough circulating insulin to keep this increase of glucose under control, the end result is higher glucose readings in the morning. To help deal with this, be sure to eat breakfast every day, because doing so tells your body to turn off these problematic hormones. Try exercising later in the day. You may need a medication adjustment to target the morning glucose.

Disasters

During the aftermath of Hurricane Katrina, thousands of people with diabetes were stranded without medication and supplies for many days, resulting in medical emergencies. That's why disaster planning is an important part of self-care. Keep a backpack full of all of the equipment you'd need for at least 2 weeks in a safe and secure location. Include a waterproof and insulated kit for testing supplies, medications, prescription numbers (especially handy if they are from a national pharmacy chain, so they can be filled throughout the country), and copies of medical information. Mark your calendar so you know to check the expiration dates of these supplies every 6 months. Learn more at www.cdc.gov/diabetes/news/docs/disasters.htm.

Exercise

Right after exercise, you may see a temporary increase in glucose values. This happens because the liver releases its stored glucose to help your muscles keep working. Do not get discouraged if you see slight blood glucose elevation after a workout. Your numbers over the next 24 hours will be in a better range than if you hadn't exercised. Also, be on the lookout for lows several hours after finishing exercising. This is when the liver takes glucose out of the bloodstream to replenish its glucose storage.

Medication effectiveness

When your blood glucose levels come into the target range, a unique problem can arise: Your medication becomes more effective, which puts you at greater risk for blood glucose lows. If you think that this is happening to you, call your health-care provider to discuss lowering your medication dosage.

Overtreating lows

If you have personally experienced a low, you know the panic feeling that accompanies it. One gentleman reported he treated his lows by sticking his head in the fridge (with his fanny sticking out—nice visual), and eating everything in sight. Overtreating lows can cause hyperglycemia, increased calories, and, thus, weight gain. What about having a hypoglycemia kit handy (with 15 grams of glucose, and a snack to eat afterward)?

Pain

Are you in pain right now? People with diabetes do have higher rates of pain. (You are probably tired of hearing the "people with diabetes have higher rates of" x, y, and z, but my job is to keep you informed so you know your options.) Pain—whether short or long term—can raise blood glucose levels. It also interferes with everyday life and one's ability to perform diabetes self-care behaviors. A decreased enjoyment in life can lead to distress and depression. Ending this association of pain and depression may require the use of medication (painkillers) and cognitive behavioral therapy (a method of dealing with the negative thoughts typically related to pain, as facilitated by a medical social worker or psychologist). Pain is subjective. Have a candid talk about it with your health-care provider to get a plan on how to make it better.

Somogyi effect

The Somogyi effect, also known as rebound hyperglycemia, is a pattern of undetected blood glucose lows followed by highs (hyperglycemia). This most often happens in the middle of the night and is caused by insulin or diabetes pills working too well, sending blood glucose levels way down. To counteract this imbalance, the liver releases its stored glucose. The end result is that blood glucose levels can swing too high in the other direction.

If you are waking up with high blood glucose readings and are wondering whether you're experiencing the Somogyi effect, set your alarm between 2 and 3 a.m. and check your blood glucose (sigh!). It takes detective work to figure out what made the glucose plummet and your care team can help. Is it too much medication? Not enough bedtime snack?

Steroids

If you have ever suffered from bursitis, arthritis, or other inflammatory issues and received a shot of cortisone or other steroid treatment, you know how helpful steroids are. But they also can raise blood glucose levels for several days after receiving treatment. Depending on the amount of steroids needed, please monitor your glucose carefully as you may also need to temporarily increase your diabetes medication, even by significant doses. Work with your health-care provider accordingly.

Stress and illness

Stress has negative effects on the body and can raise blood glucose levels. Stress can also arise in seemingly happy occasions: vacation, travel, weddings, family gatherings, retirement, and winning the lottery. If you get a high number that just doesn't make sense, take a step back and examine your stress level. Search out ways to reduce and cope with the stress in your life. Impending or actual illness can raise your glucose levels. Check your glucose often whenever you do not feel well to make sure you are okay even though that may be the last thing you want to do.

PERSONAL GOAL

Date: _____ I will:

☐ Have a hearty bedtime snack (piece of toast with peanut butter, cottage cheese, or yogurt or some nuts and a small piece of cheese).

☐ Eat breakfast most days of the week.

☐ Set the alarm for 2–3 a.m. and check my glucose.

☐ Notice my glucose patterns for 24 hours after I exercise.

☐ Have a conversation about any pain I am experiencing and ask whether a pain specialist is needed.

☐ Note pain levels in my blood glucose logbook to identify trends.

☐ Take my painkiller medication before my pain is severe.

☐ Pack an emergency–disaster supply kit in a backpack or suitcase with wheels that has at least 2 weeks' worth of medication, glucose tablets, at least 1 gallon of water, test strips, an extra glucose meter, a large box of saltine crackers, a jar of peanut butter, a small box of powdered milk, dry cereal, packages of cheese and crackers, utensils, cans of tuna, nuts, socks, underwear, a sweatsuit, and a battery-operated radio.

☐ Other: _____.

Even a psychic couldn't explain my wacky glucose readings.

WEEK
7

Socked Away

Foot safety starts with glucose control, proper hygiene, and your socks.

What are the best kinds of socks?

Cotton socks are comfortable but tend to retain moisture close to the skin, which can make your feet sweat. Sweaty feet can lead to blisters and worse. Now there are cotton-synthetic blends that pull moisture away from the feet and can prevent blisters. Synthetic fibers include acrylic, Duraspun, ionized copper, Lycra, nylon, polyester, and X-Static. Keep this in mind when you pick up your next pair. You don't need to get expensive, special socks – just know that proper fitting ones help to prevent problems and that if you are having issues, some specialty products may be of use.

What Should I Look For When Buying Socks?
- Comfort and a good deal!
- Cotton-synthetic blends for exercising.
- Seamless socks for leisure time (material is less important).
- For dressy occasions, consider microfiber acrylic alternatives.
- Check the fabric content.
- Avoid constricting bands.
- Look for wide-fit socks if you have swollen ankles.
- If you are prone to infections, look for ones with copper or silver or antibacterial listed on the tag.
- Be wary of the quality of "diabetic socks" sold at a dollar store.
- Your local pharmacy may carry specialty socks. You can also visit these stores on the web:
    - The Diabetic Sock Store at www.diabeticsockstore.com; 866-848-9327
    - Foot Smart at www.footsmart.com; 800-707-9928
    - Smooth Toe at www.smoothtoe-socks.com; 888-573-5277

Glucose checkup

In the past week, what was your highest blood glucose level? _____ mg/dL

The lowest? _____ mg/dL

Why? _____

PERSONAL GOAL

Date: _____ I will:

☐ Take inventory: discard socks with holes or knee-high nylons that fall down (they can bunch up and create blisters).
☐ Invest in my feet through good-fitting socks.
☐ Check my local pharmacy for diabetic socks.
☐ Visit websites that carry safe socks.
☐ Other: _____.

 Now I need to diversify my sock options.

Incretin Mimetics

Incretin mimetics are a relatively new class of drugs that mimic or enhance the naturally occurring gut hormone, glucagon-like peptide-1 (GLP-1).

Huh? Okay, when food passes through the intestine, special cells in the lower gut release an incretin hormone, called GLP-1 (just to make it easy to remember). People with diabetes often lack sufficient amounts of both hormones, GLP-1 and insulin. This GLP-1 hormone (taken by injection) makes the pancreas release insulin only when glucose is high. This class of drugs is effective in reducing glucose and weight. Yes, there is a bonus: People drop about 6 pounds on average after 6 months of taking incretins.

Types of GLP-1 Injections

Brand name (generic name)	Dosage	Timing	Average weight loss	Average A1C (glucose) drop in 6 months
Exenatide (Byetta)	5 or 10 micrograms	Twice daily, within 60 minutes before breakfast and dinner	6 pounds	0.8% (or 22 mg/dL)
Liraglutide (Victoza)*	0.6 milligrams daily for one week: if not effective, increase to 1.2 milligrams for 1 week; if still not effective, increase to 1.8 milligrams	Daily, regardless of mealtime	7–8 pounds	1.1–1.5% (24–33 mg/dL)
Long-acting exenatide (Bydureon)	2 milligrams	Every 7 days, regardless of mealtime, injected immediately after powder is mixed	6 pounds	1.3% (28 mg/dL)

*Not advisable for those with a personal or family history of multiple endocrine neoplasia type 2 diabetes, as well as medullary thyroid carcinoma.

Fun fact: Incretins were derived after decades of research looking into the saliva of the Gila monster (a slow-moving lizard native to the southwestern U.S. that eats about four times per year). Don't worry—it is made in laboratories, not taken from lizards, so it's fine for people to use. The lizard's saliva contains a protein called exendin-4, which works like the hormone GLP-1, but it lasts longer in the body. Both GLP-1 and exendin-4 cause the pancreas to release more insulin in response to meals, which helps control blood glucose levels.

Possible side effects or considerations

GLP-1 injections have the following possible side effects:
- Nausea is common at first. Nausea decreases after meal.
- Exenatide only: Do not take if you skip a meal; do not take after a meal (may cause vomiting).
- Low glucose can occur when used in combination with insulin or with pills listed in the Oral Medications table in Day 12, under Insulin secretagogues.
- Prescribed for people with type 2 diabetes, although, according to an article published in *Diabetes Care,* people with type 1 diabetes may also benefit from incretins (as they give the insulin-producing beta-cells a boost).
- Do not mix in the same injection with insulin.
- Not recommended for people with severe kidney problems, high triglycerides, digestion problems, or family history of thyroid cancer.
- Check package insert for storage and discard instructions. For example, the exenatide prefilled pen you are using may be kept at room temperature, not to exceed 77°F (but keep the unopened ones in the refrigerator at 36–46°F); discard pen 30 days after first use, even if the pen still has some medication in it. Store Victoza for 30 days at 59–86°F.
- Be sure to rotate sites. Give that one favorite injection spot a rest.

PERSONAL GOAL

Date: _____ I will:

☐ Increase my Victoza as directed.

☐ Bring my Byetta pen with me and inject it anytime within 60 minutes before breakfast and dinner (as prescribed).

☐ Mark on my calendar 28 days after starting a new Byetta pen so I can remember when to start a new one.

☐ Mark on my calendar or set my phone to remind me to take my weekly Bydureon injection every 7 days.

☐ Dispose of my used needles according to local laws and regulations.

☐ Report episodes of hypoglycemia or severe nausea to my health-care provider.

☐ Other: _____.

 I give my pet Gila monster lemon wedges, and still no Byetta!

Exercise Fundamentals

When is the best time to exercise?

The best time for exercise is when you're most likely to do it. Many people prefer to get their exercise done first thing in the morning; others prefer after work. Try to pick a time that fits your schedule and works for you.

Do I need a pre-exercise snack?

Some people do require a pre-exercise snack. It depends on your blood glucose level at the time, the planned physical activity, when you had your last meal, and the intensity of the workout. Consider having a pre-exercise snack to prevent hypoglycemia if you take insulin secretagogues (see Day 12 and the pills described in the table Oral Medications) or insulin, *and*—

- Your glucose is less than 100 mg/dL.
- You will exercise before a meal.
- You will be active for more than 30 minutes (especially if more than an hour).

Based on a 150-pound person, you'd need about 30–40 grams of carbohydrate snack for 1 hour of activity. If you plan on 30 minutes, you'd need 15–20 grams of carbohydrate.

Warm up your engine

Warming up prepares your body for increased activity by bringing oxygen into your muscles. It reduces risk for injury. Do 5 minutes of warm-up activities, such as knee lifts, arm windmills, gentle jumping jacks, or walking or slowly jogging in place.

Exercise and Glucose Levels

If you take insulin or insulin secretagogues (see the Oral Medications table in Day 12), check your blood glucose before exercise.

Yes, it's a pain and it's inconvenient. But it can save you from feeling lousy for hours from an unexpected low glucose and potential injury (including to others if you get behind a wheel and you go low). Carry rapid-acting sugar (like glucose tablets, hard candy, or sugary drinks) in case of a low. Suggested glucose levels are as follows:

- Right before exercise: 120 mg/dL or higher.
- During: check every 30 minutes; glucose should be at or above 100 mg/dL to resume exercise. If not, treat for low.
- After exercise: Glucose should be within target established by you and your health-care provider.

Stretch it

After a brief warm-up, another 5 minutes of stretching makes the exercise more comfortable. Stretch slowly, and don't bounce or hold your breath. Go from head-to-toe with gentle movements to stretch your neck, shoulders, back, legs, ankles, and feet.

Move it!

If you haven't been getting much physical activity recently, you'll need to start slowly and with realistic goals. Give yourself time to build up. Start with 5 minutes a day. After a week of that, go up to 10

More Glucose Tips

- If glucose is less than 70 mg/dL, treat the low, and wait to exercise for a few hours. If it is 71–100 mg/dL, have a snack.
- If you have type 1 diabetes and your glucose is above 250 mg/dL, check for ketones. Continue exercise if your ketones are negative.
- If you have type 2 diabetes and feel well, you can exercise with glucose less than 300 mg/dL.
- If you exercise for extended periods of time, check your glucose every 30 minutes during exercise, and hourly for a few hours after you finish exercising.
- Carry snacks to replenish energy burned or to treat for lows.

minutes a day. Continue ramping up until you're getting at least 150 minutes per week.

For the best health benefits, strive for 30 minutes of moderate activity on most days, such as walking briskly, golfing (carry or pull the clubs), hiking, gardening, bicycling, weight training, and light aerobic workouts.

Cool off!

Cool down after exercising by doing 5 minutes of slow walking or stretches.

Check your blood glucose after exercise

Checking your blood glucose after exercise helps you take any action to prevent lows, and it lets you know whether you're safe to drive.

Stay hydrated

When you exercise, your body needs more fluid to keep it cool. Drink water before, during, and after exercise to prevent dehydration.

What exercise factors can affect my glucose?

The following exercise factors can affect glucose levels:
- Your level of fitness. The less fit you are, the greater the impact exercise will have on your blood glucose levels. This means as you get in shape, your exercise-related blood glucose fluctuations should decrease.
- The type of exercise you do. If you do only one type of exercise, you will see an increased effect on your blood glucose levels if you try a different type of exercise. For example, if you jog routinely and then start swimming, the swimming will have a bigger effect on blood glucose levels.
- Your pre-exercise blood glucose level.
- Whether you drank alcohol the previous day.
- Whether you exercised the previous day, which can have a lasting effect.
- Your hydration state.

Exercise improves insulin sensitivity (whether it's your own or the insulin you inject), heart function, muscle mass, and weight management. What are you willing to change to make that happen?

PERSONAL GOAL

Date: _____ I will:

☐ Check my blood glucose level if I feel nervous, shaky, or hungry during my workout or several hours after and treat for lows if it's less than 70 mg/dL.

☐ Check my blood glucose level, have a 15- to 20-gram carbohydrate snack before activity, and recheck my blood glucose level afterward. I will adjust my snack size until my before and after blood glucose levels are similar.

☐ Drink a glass of water 30 minutes before and after I exercise.

☐ Schedule an appointment to exercise when I'm least likely to cancel it.

☐ Squeeze in a 10-minute break for a brisk walk.

☐ Warm up for 5 minutes by doing gentle jumping jacks or walking in place.

☐ Download the stellar smartphone app, Nike Training (has interactive plans, including sections: Get Lean, Get Toned, Get Strong, and Get Focused).

☐ Other: _____.

My pancreas is smiling—I took a 30-minute brisk walk.

Coffee and Cigarettes

Cup of Joe

Enjoying a cup of coffee is perfectly fine as long as you don't add a ton of sugar and cream. If you don't know the nutrient contents of your favorite coffee drinks, prepare yourself. Some of those specialty drinks have the same amount of calories, fat, and carbohydrates as a fast-food meal.

What about tea?

Aside from caffeine (tea generally has less caffeine than coffee or soda) and cream-and-sugar issues, tea provides many health benefits and does not pose a problem for people with diabetes.

Smoking: It gets in more than just your eyes

Would you be outraged if someone slipped a drug into your bloodstream without your permission? Nonsmokers, beware! This happens every time you inhale secondhand smoke. Walk around most outdoor public areas and you'll likely encounter plumes of cigarette smoke from people mingling in corridors or hovering around entranceways. You're breathing in toxins. So much for trying to get out for some fresh air!

What can you do? Be on the lookout for cigarette smoke and try to avoid it. Short of holding your breath, make a plan to get away from it. What if your partner smokes? Decide what you are willing to accept and negotiate the rest. Your health is on the line. It's one thing if someone else decides to smoke—it's their body—but it's quite a different issue if they turn you into a passive smoker.

What a drag.

For years, the Surgeon General has said that smoking is hazardous to your health. As obvious as that sounds, many smokers are unaware of the basic dangers they face. People who have diabetes and smoke are 11 times more likely to have a heart attack than those who have diabetes and don't smoke.

Ready for more? Smoking increases the risks for blindness, kidney disease, impotence, amputation, tooth loss (more than 40% of people over age 65 years who smoke lose their teeth), bad breath, and facial wrinkling. The same goes for cigar and pipe smokers. If that's not enough, think about what nicotine exposure does to a fetus or newborn: It increases the chances for obesity and diabetes later in life.

Ready to put out the fire?

Quitting smoking is not easy, but researchers have found a method that works well.

1. Make a list of reasons why you want to quit (e.g., for your health, your kids, save hundreds of dollars).
2. Pick a quitting date and stick to it. Plan how you will fight the urge to smoke (e.g., go for a walk, go out a different door, don't hang out with smokers). Ask your health-care provider to recommend a prescription (combining the nicotine patch with the drug Zyban is nearly 90% effective).
3. Change your habits. If you smoke on the porch in a comfortable chair, smoke standing up. Don't smoke while driving (have a smoke-free car). Smoke alone (it's not as fun as smoking with the gang). Figure out what triggers your desire for a cigarette.
4. Prepare your environment to quit. Get rid of ashtrays and lighters. Wash your clothes, so they don't smell like smoke. Buy only a single pack at a time, not a carton. Tap into a support system (many hospitals offer free smoking-cessation classes). Ask your smoking pals to not offer you cigarettes.

PERSONAL GOAL

Date: _____ I will:

☐ Find out how many carbohydrates and calories are in my favorite cappuccino, latte, or specialty coffee drink.

☐ Learn how my cappuccino changes my blood glucose.

☐ Pick a day to quit smoking.

☐ Request help from my health-care provider, so I can kick the smoking habit.

☐ Get help quitting smoking by calling 1-800-NO-BUTTS or 1-800-QUIT-NOW.

☐ Calculate how much money I'll save by cutting out lattes or cigarettes.

☐ Other: _____.

 Make me a secondhand smoker only if I can make you a secondhand diabetic.

MONTH 2: REVIEW

Date: _____

Congratulations on making it through 2 months of intensive diabetes self-management. Take a minute to reflect and rate your progress.

Please circle the answer that best represents your assessment of the past 2 months:

CHECK NUMBERS
1. I tested my glucose:
    a. Rarely (less than 20%)
    b. Sometimes (20–80%)
    c. Mostly (more than 80%)

SOLVE PROBLEMS
2. I know to call my health-care provider when my glucose values are consistently above 250 mg/dL for 2 consecutive days or less than 70 mg/dL on any given day.
    a. Yes   b. No

EAT WISELY
3. I have found enjoyable foods that my diabetes can handle.
    a. Yes   b. No

BE ACTIVE
4. I am active for at least 30 minutes 5 days a week.
    a. Rarely (less than 20%)
    b. Sometimes (20–80%)
    c. Mostly (more than 80%)

REDUCE STRESS
5. I have tried and found new ways to deal with stress.
    a. Yes   b. No

UNDERSTAND MEDICATIONS
6. I know how my medications work.
    a. Yes   b. No

REDUCE RISKS
7. Did I do at least one of the following? Flossed my teeth daily, saw the dentist, got a flu shot, or got my kidneys checked.
    a. Yes   b. No

ADD HUMOR
8. I notice more subtle humor in situations.
    a. Yes   b. No

MONTH 3

Laughin' Langerhans

By Theresa Garnero

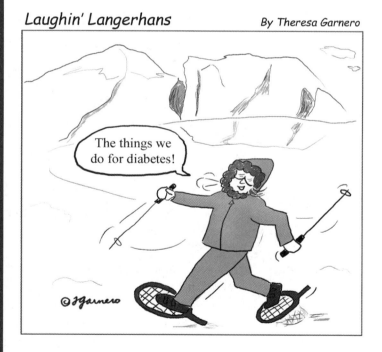

WEEK
9

Worth the Weight

Most adults are in a weight-management state of mind because the majority of us have a weight issue. Although a recent study suggests that Americans tend to be in denial about their weight, many adults said they lost weight when they actually gained! Our obsession with a quick fix to shedding pounds feeds a multibillion-dollar diet industry. We'd rather spend our hard-earned dollars on fad diets, miracle supplements, and packaged foods than look within for the solution to permanently losing weight.

The solution is figuring out your primary motivator, a concept described by Kay Laughrey, RD, and by regularly self-modulating your level of stress, according to Laurel Mellin, RD, PhD.

Change is more likely to last when the motivation comes from within. Why do you want to manage weight?

1. Better health and energy
2. Vanity (what's wrong with wanting to improve appearance?)
3. Improve well-being, self-esteem, and stress level
4. Enhance relationships
5. Save money (less medication, less eating at restaurants)
6. Fill in the blank with your reason: _____

Next, remember how these reasons connect to your life's higher purpose. That is somewhat easy—thinking about the motivation. Applying it through consistent food and activity is a challenge, especially when stressed. It is not difficult when stressed to unconsciously polish off a serving size for 10. Staying on top of weight management requires healthy everyday behaviors and staying alert to internal dialogue. When reaching for something that will work against your primary motivator for weight management, you have a split second to intervene. Are you really hungry? Is your food choice one of convenience just to get in a meal (and if so, can you eat just one portion?) or is it an attempt to quell internal stress? And what is the source of the stress? What can you do about it that doesn't involve using food as a comfort measure?

Why weight matters with diabetes

Reducing body fat improves blood glucose control. Losing weight also decreases your risk for heart disease and high blood pressure. If you are overweight, set a realistic weight-loss goal (about 1–2 pounds per week) and allow plenty of time to reach your goal. This is a new way of eating. The weight gain didn't happen overnight, and it will take even longer to come off and stay off.

Why exercise trains your fat

A single bout of exercise has short-term effects on the whole body. After only 11 days of exercise, the subcutaneous fat directly underneath the skin changes from white to brown and that's important. Called "brown adipose tissue," this brown fat helps regulate metabolism. In essence, exercise can train your fat and these fat cells can "talk" to other tissues to help with metabolism and weight management.

Why diets don't work

Diets don't work over the long term because they take the "self" out of self-care behavior. If you give your diet the power in your life, then you are not making choices; they are being made for you *by the diet*. Sure, you may see some temporary weight loss, but to maintain this loss and change eating behaviors *for life, you* have to be in the driver's seat, not your diet. Nearly 90% of dieters, or 9 of 10 people, who go on diets generally gain back the pounds they lost and then some.

How Do I Lose Weight?

Don't diet: Go on a new way of eating

There are many ways to lose weight, but great examples on how to maintain weight-management efforts can be found through the National Weight Control Registry (www.nwcr.ws), a group that studies people who have lost at least 30 pounds and kept it off for 1 year or longer. There is no single way that they all lost weight and kept it off, but certain things are common among a majority of members. Here's a short list:

- Follow a mostly low-calorie, low-fat diet.
- Eat breakfast every day.
- Weigh at least once a week.
- Watch fewer than 10 hours of television a week.
- Get an average of 1 hour of exercise per day (usually in the form of walking).

Because you have diabetes, one of the first steps you should take is to find a registered dietitian (RD), who can help you assess your diet and help you create a personalized meal plan. If you don't have an RD already, ask your health-care team about how to make this invaluable professional part of your team.

What about calories?

Calorie consumption is a major piece of the weight-management puzzle, but not the only piece (review Day 8 on how many calories you need). Of course, the amount of exercise and sleep you get play pivotal roles. Lesser-known influences on weight management are nutrient deficiencies. At a minimum, take a multivitamin daily and check with your doctor to find out whether you have enough levels of vitamin D in your system and whether you should take probiotics.

Even though it is not as simple as burning more calories than you take in, it certainly helps to understand how a few extra bites of calorie-dense food affect your effort. You've been deluged with lots of numbers. You'll have plenty of examples in week 15, but for now, you can start by getting an idea of how many calories are in some of *your* food choices—just take a gander at the label.

Food is fuel. How much fuel are you giving your body? Does your body have the engine of a Prius that only needs enough gas to drive for 30 minutes, but instead you are filling it up like it's a Hummer heading out on a road trip? To start losing weight (or stop gaining pounds), you'll need to make sure your gas tank gets only the amount of fuel it needs.

Where am I now?

Do you know how to determine whether you are overweight?

Body mass index (BMI) is a screening tool used measure a person's body fatness. It is calculated by taking weight in kilograms and dividing it by the square of height in meters. But you don't have to do all of that math; instead, you can just look at the table on the following page or find BMI calculators online.

Wait—People say that BMI is always wrong

The BMI originally was developed in the 1840s by the Belgian polymath (a person who has encyclopedic knowledge) Adolphe Quetelet, in his studies of social physics. Since then, it has become widely used. One chart doesn't fit all, but BMI is pretty reliable in people who are overweight or physically inactive. BMI can be less accurate for some groups of individuals. For the elderly and the very ill, bone densities and body frames can make BMI less accurate. Athletes often incorrectly are considered overweight according to BMI because they have more muscles, which weigh more than fat.

Wouldn't I be better off on a low-carb, high-protein diet?

Not exactly. Low-carb, high-protein diets are effective at helping you lose weight for up to 2 years, but they also go hand-in-hand with higher fat intake, which comes with risk. High fat intake can increase insulin resistance and lead to clogged arteries—and that's something to consider.

The other important issue to consider when it comes to low-carb, high-protein diets is that they limit the variety of healthy food choices you take in. You'd miss out on nutrient-dense foods like some vegetables, fruits, and high-fiber starches. Fiber helps lower cholesterol levels and prevents constipation.

The Importance of Meal Planning

What did you eat in the last 24 hours? Did you make any impulsive decisions about your food choices? Did you skip a meal? Having a plan for your meals is an important key to success. It's like planning for retirement. It takes a little thought, time, and investment, but down the road that meal plan will have saved your life.

A nutritionally balanced meal plan for people with diabetes may

BMI Table

Find your height in feet and inches on the left and then follow along the column until you reach your weight in pounds. The number in the box indicates your BMI.

	140	150	160	170	180	190	200	210	220	230	240	250	260	270	280	290	300
4'6"	34	36	39	41	43	45	48	51	53	56	58	60	63	65	68	70	72
4'8"	31	34	36	38	40	43	45	47	49	52	54	56	58	61	63	65	67
4'10"	29	31	34	36	38	40	42	44	46	48	50	52	54	57	59	61	63
5'	27	29	31	33	35	37	39	41	43	45	47	49	51	53	55	57	59
5'2"	26	27	29	31	33	35	37	38	40	42	44	46	48	49	51	53	55
5'4"	24	26	28	29	31	33	34	36	38	40	41	43	45	46	48	50	52
5'6"	23	24	26	27	29	31	32	34	36	37	39	40	42	44	45	47	49
5'8"	21	23	24	26	27	29	30	32	34	35	37	38	40	41	43	44	46
5'10"	20	22	23	24	26	27	29	30	32	33	35	36	37	39	40	42	43
6'	19	20	22	23	24	26	27	28	30	31	33	34	36	37	38	39	41
6'2"	18	19	21	22	23	24	26	27	28	30	31	32	33	35	36	37	39
6'4"	17	18	20	21	22	23	24	26	27	28	29	30	32	33	34	35	37
6'6"	16	17	19	20	21	22	23	24	25	27	28	29	30	31	32	34	35
6'8"	15	17	18	19	20	21	22	23	24	25	26	28	29	30	31	32	33

BMI categories

Less than 18.4 kg/m^2 = underweight
18.5 to 24.9 kg/m^2 = healthy weight
25 to 29.9 kg/m^2 = overweight
30 to 39.9 kg/m^2 = obese
Over 40 kg/m^2 = extremely obese

Do You Have Food-aholism?

Do you find yourself constantly thinking about food? Are you eating too much despite the negative consequences? Do you try to cut back on your food, but then overeat and feel consumed with guilt? For some people, these symptoms are not related to a simple lack of willpower. There is growing evidence for the idea of a "food addiction," much like we've already recognized for other drug dependencies.

Food addicts often feel out of control of their cravings and have very intense food cues. They tend to overeat, past the point of fullness, and can have an obsessive or compulsive relationship with food. Just like other addictions, eating certain foods, particularly high-fat and high-carb foods, can stimulate the reward center of the brain. In fact, fatty foods can be as addictive as cocaine according to a growing body of science! No wonder that pastry put a spell on you! Next time you catch yourself reaching for the cookie jar for the fifth time in a day, don't just berate yourself, consider the possibility of food addiction.

Check out these resources on food addiction for more information on diagnosis and treatment:

- Overeaters Anonymous: www.oa.org (505-891-2664)
- Food Addiction Institute: foodaddictioninstitute.org (941-747-1972)

help with weight management, which in turn may help people manage their diabetes! Why? Excess weight makes it more difficult for the body to use its limited supply of available insulin. If you are overweight, losing 7% of your weight (in many cases, just 10–15 pounds) will be the ticket to lowering blood glucose levels. Many studies show this can be accomplished by getting at least 30 minutes of exercise (this includes walking) a day and reducing calories.

You can turn things around one meal, one workout, and one food choice at a time. You've got built-in safety devices: your head, arms, and legs. Your head tells you what it wants to eat. Your legs have to take you to the food. Your arms bring the food to your mouth. Make *health-conscious* choices.

PERSONAL GOAL

Date: _____ I will:

☐ Avoid skipping breakfast and eat most of my calories before 7 p.m.

☐ Do at least one healthy thing today.

☐ Wait 15 minutes before treating myself to unhealthy snacks (even a 5-minute distraction can thwart a craving). If I can't wait, I'll have just a few bites and savor them.

☐ Brush my teeth after eating to send a message to my brain that the meal is over.

☐ Call an RD to help me get a weight-management and meal plan.

☐ Plan at least 3 days' worth of meals ahead of time this week.

☐ Start a food and activity diary to track what I eat and what activities I do.

☐ Focus my weight-management efforts by exercising 60 minutes a day to maintain my current weight or crank it up to 90 minutes a day to lose weight.

☐ Take a multivitamin.

☐ Other: _____ .

 Why can't my brain be addicted to veggies?

Fun in Function

For those of you who are exercising regularly—and for those of you who aren't—check out these ideas for inspiring physical activity. Circle at least two that you are willing to do this month.

- Walk around a park I've never visited.
- See a new exhibit in a museum.
- See how many different kinds of birds I can spot in a 30-minute walk.
- Go bowling.
- Plant something.
- Go rollerblading.
- Take a bike ride through a scenic route.
- Buy and use a hula-hoop or jump rope.
- Play golf (regular or miniature).
- Join an ultimate Frisbee league.
- Take a dance class.
- Find an exercise pal to take the "work" out of "workout."
- Walk to your next dinner date.
- Do nude yoga. Okay, do that fun hot yoga!
- Walk somewhere for a picnic.
- Saunter downtown to people watch.
- Do jumping jacks in the pool.

Why should I write down my results when my meter has a memory?

You don't have to write down your results. The benefit, however, is that on occasion, putting all the puzzle pieces together in one spot (like glucose, amount of medication taken, amount of carbs and exercise, and level of stress) helps everyone see patterns that might not be clear from simply looking in the memory. This is especially helpful for 1 week before going into your health-care provider's office, as most meters do not track all these variables. Some glucose monitor companies allow you to download their software for free but will charge you for the cable that makes it possible to use the software. Smartphone apps make this even easier (check out Glooko Logbook).

What if I don't want to use a computer?

You can use the meter company's logbook (call them to ask to mail you another paper logbook). Many people also create their own personal systems. It doesn't really matter, as long as the information is organized and you and your health-care provider can interpret the data.

Does my meter tell me my A1C?

You can use the memory averages on a regular glucose monitor to get a *general* idea about your A1C, but it's not the same as an A1C test. The chart below shows how average glucose levels correlate to A1C levels. Your health-care provider may refer to your A1C as estimated average glucose.

A1C (%)	Estimated average glucose	A1C (%)	Estimated average glucose
6	126	10	240
7	154	11	269
8	183	12	298
9	212	13	326

What was your last A1C test result?_____ Date: _____

PERSONAL GOAL

Date: _____ I will:

☐ Check out my meter's memory functions.
☐ Ask my local pharmacist or CDE about the functions on my meter.
☐ Check my blood glucose before and 2 hours after breakfast or another meal.
☐ Ask someone to help me set up my software program.
☐ Print out a copy of my recent blood glucose values.
☐ Keep a consistent, organized record of my blood glucose values.
☐ Other: _____.

Thanks to A1C goals,
I can strive to be below average.

WEEK
11

Blood Pressure Medications

Diabetes and high blood pressure are siblings fighting for your attention. If your blood pressure is above 140/80 mmHg, you are at risk for cardiovascular complications (the big ones: heart attack and stroke).

An underappreciated mechanism occurs with high blood glucose levels. Most know that it causes sugar to pile up *outside* of the cell. This area of higher concentration pulls water from the cell and into the bloodstream. The fluid has nowhere to go and since it is in a closed blood vessel system, the blood pressure increases. Certainly, there are hereditary factors to high blood pressure, so even though your glucose level may return to ideal, blood pressure may not. And then there is our passion for salt intake, which only worsens the situation by causing fluid to stay in the blood vessels. It is critical to get the blood pressure close to 140/80 mmHg. You may "feel fine" and try to negotiate with your doctor for months to lower it with diet and exercise. Please don't wait too long to take action. Taking blood pressure medications can extend your lease on life. This is a summary of many available blood pressure meds. Many more combination forms exist.

Types of blood pressure medicines	Brand name (generic name)	Possible side effects or issues
Angiotensin-Converting Enzyme (ACE) Inhibitors (lowers blood pressure, reduces insulin resistance, protects the lining of blood vessels and kidneys; one of the first choices for treating hypertension)	**Accupril** (quinapril) **Altace** (ramipril) **Capoten** (captopril) **Lotensin** (benazepril) **Mavik** (trandolapril) **Prinivil** (lisinopril) **Vasotec** (enalapril) **Zestril** (lisinopril)	*May* cause a cough, although that is a positive sign that the harmful chemicals that narrow blood vessels are being blocked. You may not have a cough and this medicine still works effectively. May aid in the prevention of diabetes and of diabetic kidney disease. A rare, but serious condition can occur with swelling in the tongue and mouth. It can also cause high levels of potassium. Do not take salt substitutes or potassium without talking to a doctor. Do not use if pregnant.
Angiotensin II Receptor Blockers (ARBs) (effects are similar to those of ACE inhibitors)	**Atacand** (candesartanl) **Avapro** (irbesartan) **Benicar** (olmesartan) **Cozaar** (losartan) **Diovan** (valsartan) **Edarbi** (azilsartan) **Micardis** (telmisartan)	Blocks harmful chemicals that can narrow blood vessels without the coughing sometimes seen with ACE inhibitors. As a result, ARBs are more expensive. May cause dizziness and upset stomach (olmesartan can cause severe intestinal symptoms). Do not use salt substitutes or potassium without talking to a doctor. Do not use if pregnant. May aid in the prevention of diabetic kidney disease. Several guidelines recommend that people with diabetes who have heart or blood vessel disease, congestive heart failure, or protein in the urine be prescribed an ACE inhibitor or ARB, even if they don't have high blood pressure.

Types of blood pressure medicines	Brand name (generic name)	Possible side effects or issues
Calcium Channel Blockers (CCBs) (blocks calcium in the heart vessels, which makes the arteries relax and allows more oxygen in)	**Adalat** (nifedipine) **Calan SR** (verapamil ER) **Cardizem** (diltiazem) **Norvasc** (amlodipine) **Plendil** (felodipine) **Procardia** (nifedipine)	May cause swelling in the hands or feet, constipation, upset stomach, or flushed skin. Call your doctor if you feel short of breath, have any swelling, or feel your heart has skipped beats.
Alpha-Blockers (relaxes the heart vessels and slows down the heart)	**Cardura** (doxazosin) **Hytrin** (terazosin) **Minipress** (prazosin)	May cause sudden dizziness if you get up too fast, especially with the first few doses. Do not suddenly stop taking alpha-blockers.
Beta-Blockers (relaxes blood vessels and helps the heart beat regularly; also used for chest pain)	**Inderal** (propranolol) **Tenormin** (atenolol) **Toprol** (metoprolol)	Helps the heart work more easily. Some risky side effects are as follows: may block your ability to detect hypoglycemia, increase insulin resistance, and worsen diabetes control. Some experience depression, nightmares, and insomnia.
Hydrochloro-thiazides (known as a water pill or thiazide diuretic; relaxes small blood vessels)	HCTZ	Inexpensive and used in combination with many types of blood pressure pills. For doses above 12.5 milligrams, some may experience cramps, rashes, and loss of potassium.
Combination: **Alpha- and Beta-Blockers** (see descriptions above)	**Coreg** (carvedilol)	Lowers insulin resistance. May cause sudden dizziness when standing up. May cause upset stomach and mask signs of low blood glucose.
Combination: **ACE** or **ARB** plus diuretic	**ALL ARBs and most ACE are available with HCTZ.** **Exforge HCT** (valsartan and amlodipine and HCTZ) **Edarbyclor** (azilsartan/ chlorthalidone)	Good option for chronic renal insufficiency.

Types of blood pressure medicines	Brand name (generic name)	Possible side effects or issues
Combination: **ACE** or **ARB** plus **CCB**	**Exforge** (valsartan and amlodipine) **Lexxel** (enalapril and felodipine) **Lotrel** (amlodipine and benazepril) **Tarka** (trandolapril and verapamil ER**)** **Tribenzor** (olmesartan, amlodipine, and hydrocholorothiazide**)**	Additive blood pressure reduction. Report swelling or edema.
Combination: **Thiazide** plus **Beta-Blocker**	**Atenolol/HTCZ** **Corzide** (nadolol and bendroflume-thiazide) **Inderide** (propranolol and HCTZ) **Ziac** (bisoprolol and HCTZ)	Additive blood pressure reduction. Thiazides improve beta-blocker efficacy in African Americans. Fatigue, sexual dysfunction, glucose intolerance may be an issue.
Combination: **Renin inhibitor** plus **CCB** and **Thiazide**	**Amturnide** (aliskiren and amlodipine and HCTZ)	Report swelling or edema. Some common reactions include facial flushing, heart palpitations, fatigue, and skin reactions.
Combination: **ARB** plus **CCB** and **Thiazide**	**Exforge HCT** (valsartan and amlodipine and HCTZ) **Tribenzor** (olmesartan and amlodipine and HCTZ)	Report swelling or edema. Some common side effects include sore throat, head or chest cold, dizziness, tiredness, muscle spasms, and indigestion.

Is it a good thing to know my doctor's number by heart?

WEEK

12

 Groupies Have Lower Glucose

Get support. Study after study has shown a strong link between having a support system and effective diabetes management.

Why?

When your support system cares for you and cares about your health, it is motivating. You don't feel alone and you are more likely to make positive changes in your self-care regimen if you have a strong support system. Your family and friends can play a pivotal supporting role in your diabetes care, but outside support groups can be just as (or even more) helpful.

Consider a diabetes support group

Support groups provide opportunities for you to meet other people with diabetes in an informal atmosphere to discuss anything related to diabetes in a nonthreatening environment. You can talk about the impact diabetes has on your life, ask others about their successful strategies, and get support for healthy living. It helps to be connected with someone who is in a similar situation.

What to Look for in a Support Group

- *Location.* Is transportation an issue?
- *Time.* Does the group's schedule match with yours?
- *Leader.* Who leads the group: a health-care professional or someone with diabetes?
- *Dynamics.* Is the group's age-range, culture, ethnicity, language, and type of diabetes a good fit for you?
- *Participation.* Do you have an opportunity to interact?
- *Perception.* Did you think your first meeting helped or not? Do you want to go back? When in doubt, give the group a second chance.

Where can I find a diabetes support group?

You can ask your health-care provider, local hospital, diabetes education program, library, or church. Now that the 2013 American Diabetes Association's National Standards for Diabetes Self-Management Education and Support emphasize the critical importance for ongoing support, we hope to see funding for programs to fill this need. The Internet is another place to check (Week 21 covers the diabetes online community, but if you need to jump in now, visit www.dlife.com, www.diabeticconnect.com, or www.diabetesdaily.com).

PERSONAL GOAL

Date: _____ I will:

☐ Locate and attend a diabetes support group.
☐ Ask my partner to attend a class or support group with me.
☐ Talk to someone who will be supportive about my diabetes.
☐ Contact the American Diabetes Association at
   1-800-DIABETES (1-800-342-2383) to find a local
   diabetes support group.
☐ Other: _____.

 My friends help me get by and get into trouble.

WEEK
13

 Communicating with Your Health-Care Team

Have you ever walked out of a medical appointment and wondered what was just said? Sometimes doctors or other providers seem so busy, use words you don't understand, or ask questions you don't want to answer, and talking with them may make you feel confused, overwhelmed, or even guilty. This isn't because they are uncaring people, but usually it's a result of a clash of wording and ways of understanding your disease. Many people feel some anxiety when going to the doctor's office. Emotions are probably heightened because you know you will talk about your diabetes, which is personal and important. Having a strategy prepared before your medical appointment is helpful.

How can I get the most out of my clinic visits?

Preparation. First, think of a friend or family member who can come with you to your appointment. Someone who you trust, who knows a bit about your diabetes, and who can help you stay calm is the best fit. This person can help you advocate for your needs and take notes during the appointment so you can remember what you talked about.

Second, make a list of questions and concerns that you would like addressed and include a list of medications that need refilling (check your supply of medications, insulin, and test strips). Have you realized you need to see a specialist, like an ophthalmologist, while reading this book? Add that to your list; your health-care team probably will have recommended providers for you with whom they can coordinate.

Your AAA rescue team: ask, advocate, assert

It is important to remember that you are in charge of your diabetes care, regardless of any intimidation you may feel at the doctor's office. If you don't understand something your doctor says or you don't know why you're being told to take a certain medication or test your blood glucose at a certain time, ASK!

Advocating for your needs is a critical component to navigating the health-care system, whether it comes to insurance, prescription costs, scheduling appointments, or getting the care you need. Communicating with your health-care team involves compromising. You try to learn how to fit into their language and culture, and they try to fit in yours.

Tips for Health Care Visits

Be prepared for your visits by following these tips:
- Prepare a list of questions you want answered.
- Bring your blood glucose logbook (best if you bring a printout or photo-copied form).
- Provide a list of all medications, their doses, and any herbal supplements you're taking.
- Complete a 2- or 3-day food diary to share during your visit.

During the visit:
- Bring something in case you have to wait (e.g., a book or crossword puzzle).
- Bring along a friend or relative to help you remember all that was said and done.
- Be honest!
- Ask for printed materials or written instructions.

After the visit:
- Call if you need clarification about anything.
- Follow through with your health-care provider's instructions.

You are the most important person on the diabetes care team. Take an active role in your health to maximize the quality of care you receive.

PERSONAL GOAL

Date: _____ I will:

☐ Ask a friend or family member to accompany me to my next doctor's appointment.

☐ Reflect on what went well and what I'd like to change from my last doctor's appointment.

☐ Start a list of topics to bring up at my next appointment.

☐ Write down any part of my diabetes regimen that I don't understand.

☐ Other: _____.

MONTH 3: REVIEW

Date: _____

Three months have passed since picking up this book. Reflect on the self-care behaviors and jot down what is working well and what could use a little work. No judgment here.

Enter my weight: _____

Self-care behavior	Working well	Needs some effort
Eat wisely		
Be active		
Check numbers		
Understand medications		
Reduce stress		
Reduce risks		
Solve problems		
Add humor		

MONTH 4

Laughin' Langerhans By *Theresa Garnero*

"You've been randomly selected for additional screening."

WEEK
14

 Your Exercise Map

Copy this chart to keep track of your weekly physical activity.

Week of: _____

Day	Glucose before	Glucose after	Exercise type (aerobic, resistance, stretch)	Notes
Mon				
Tues				
Wed				
Thurs				
Fri				
Sat				
Sun				

Source: Adapted with permission from *Exercise Manual: an Exercise Guide for Adults with Diabetes*, 2nd ed., by Richard Peng, MS, MBA, ACSM-RCEP, CDE.

Tired of the parakeet chirping, "Exercise for 30 minutes a day"? How about this?

A recent study looked at non-exercising people who started a walking program. It compared the number of steps taken per day and minutes spent walking and their health outcomes. The number of steps per day was associated with protection against certain health problems (such as hypertension, cancer, stroke, and depressive symptoms). By contrast, time spent walking was associated with protection against one health problem, hypertension.

> If you don't have enough time or the ability to engage in physical activity of at least moderate intensity, go accumulate steps! They add up and can prevent health problems.

Take comfort in knowing your physical activity efforts are worth it. Whether you build up steps in your daily activities or get out for a chunk of time to move your body. Go for it!

PERSONAL GOAL

Date: _____ I will:

☐ Record my physical activity for 1 week.
☐ Compare how I feel and what happens to my glucose when I get 30 minutes of exercise versus 3,000 steps in a day.
☐ Buy that pedometer to measure my daily steps.
☐ Other: _____.

 I am capable of unconditional steps.

Work Yourself Sick?

Do you have a lot of job-related stress? If you do, you need to learn how to manage it. People with high levels of work-related stress have 50% more health-care expenses, according to a National Institute of Occupational Safety and Health report. Your ability to handle work stress can affect your diabetes management.

Stress on the job comes from ourselves (our personalities and work habits) and the work environment (support from peers and management, job expectations, work hours, and physical demands). We work hard, work for longer hours, and have crazy commutes. One study found that people who had shorter commutes and lower salaries were happier and less stressed than those with longer commutes and higher salaries. The time not spent on commuting allowed time for extra sleep, relaxation, and connecting with friends.

Techniques to De-stress Your Work Life

- Turn gripes into gratitude. Complaining is commonplace, so turn it around and look for the positives. Replace "I had the worst day ever" with "The best thing that happened to me today was . . . " Look for things that bring you joy.

- Beat the clock. Running late to work can stress out anyone. Turn that situation around by leaving early for work, so you'll have time to leisurely commute. Look around as you go to work; you'll see things you never saw for years.

- Organize, don't agonize. Tackle that tough assignment first and you won't spend days obsessing over deadlines. Budget time for projects like you would your money for household bills. Get a spending plan—for your work time. Prioritize and evaluate your goals daily.

- Manage your technology time. Set up a general schedule to check e-mails at the start of your day, midway through, and an hour before leaving. Manage your phone time by screening calls. Return calls before lunch or close to quitting time to keep conversations short.

- One pile at a time. Multitasking can be great, but it's a problem if you never get anything done. Tackle projects one at a time, if you can.

- Take a break. Get away from the work. Go get a glass of water or a cup of tea. Find a few minutes to close your eyes and visualize your favorite getaway.

- Stash healthy snacks. People who are stressed out tend to eat to cope with that stress. People who experience job-related stress are 73% more likely to become obese. Stock up on healthy desk snacks, so you stack your chances for better productivity and glucose.
- Find the funny. Find someone who is willing to laugh and share humorous anecdotes.
- Control what you can. Learn as you go and decide what to let go.
- Beware of burnout. If you dread going to work, is it a matter of needing some personal time or do you need to plan for a different path to bring you joy in your work?

PERSONAL GOAL

Date: _____ I will:

☐ Put in that long-overdue request for a vacation.
☐ Identify three good things that happened every day this week.
☐ Take a daily break.
☐ Block off time to finish that one project that's been nagging me.
☐ Buy an assortment of tasty healthy snacks.
☐ Other: _____.

 Pardon me for playing hooky today.

WEEK
15

The Art of Travel

Is it time to recharge the batteries with a long-deserved vacation or are you headed out on a business trip? A little planning goes a long way to ensuring that diabetes doesn't interfere with your travel plans.

Before you go

If you know you are going on a long trip, you may want to get a checkup about 1 month before you leave. Ask your doctor about immunizations (if you are traveling abroad), how to adjust medications with time-zone changes (when five or fewer time zones are crossed, no change is required, but more than that, get advice), and what to do if you get ill on your trip. Also ask for an extra prescription for diabetes medications and glucose-monitoring supplies (keep these with you at all times during travel), so if your luggage is misplaced or stolen, you will have an easier time getting your diabetes supplies replaced.

What should I pack?

Always carry diabetes supplies and medications in your carry-on luggage (with your medications in a separate clear bag) along with some favorite, hearty snacks. Doing this will save you the hassle if food isn't so great and can save your life if your luggage is lost. Also, the extreme temperatures in the luggage compartment in airplanes can damage medications. Whenever possible, bring prescription labels for medication and medical devices (not required by the Transportation Security Administration, but it can make the screening process go more smoothly).

Things to Pack

- Medications (and insulin) with their original pharmacy or prescription labels. Make sure the labels match the name on your airline ticket
- Blood glucose monitor and supplies (make sure lancets are capped)
- Twice the amount of diabetes supplies you think you might need
- Glucose tablets, if you are at risk for going low
- Snacks (crackers with cheese or peanut butter, protein bars, or nuts)
- Socks and shoes that won't cause blisters
- Medical insurance cards
- Emergency phone numbers, including your health-care team
- Medical alert bracelet, especially if you take diabetes medication or insulin
- Insulated bag to keep insulin or other injectable medications cool
- Water
- Sunscreen

At the airport

Arrive early. Notify the security screener that you have diabetes and that you are carrying your supplies with you. If you have trouble getting through security, ask for a supervisor to assist you. If you are wearing an insulin pump, ask for a visual inspection. Advise the screener that it cannot be removed because it is attached to a catheter under your skin. Furthermore, note that full-body or X-ray scanners used for airport security screening may affect the function of insulin pump or continuous glucose monitoring (CGM) devices. Although not required, people with diabetes can present a travel letter obtained from their physicians to avoid possible damage caused by exposure to imaging equipment in airports. The motor of an insulin delivery pump or glucose monitoring device may experience electromagnetic malfunctioning when passed through an airport security scanner. However, little research has been published on the potential impact of that exposure, so it is best to be safe. If traveling alone, consider telling at least one person you have diabetes.

PERSONAL GOAL

Date: _____ I will:

☐ Schedule an appointment for a checkup 1 month before leaving on a long trip.

☐ Ask my health-care provider for an extra diabetes medication prescription in case I need it while traveling.

☐ Make sure the prescription label is visible on all my diabetes medications.

☐ Get a translated diabetes-medical alert card (available in many languages).

☐ Carry diabetes medicines and meter supplies with me along with my medical alert bracelet.

☐ Visit www.tsa.gov to check on the latest security screening requirements.

☐ Bring a list of emergency contact phone numbers and put key contact numbers in my cell phone.

☐ Write down a list of all of my medications and pack it in my carry-on luggage.

☐ Agree to talk with a pharmacist in the country I'm visiting if I have any issues with my meds (they may have options).

 All this planning for a trip makes me want to take another vacation.

The Cost of Junk Food

Before you go after the jugular of that Danish (or any other "I know I shouldn't have" type food), think about how much "activity" it will take to "cover" those calories. During times of stress, boredom, or at moments when tempting unhealthy treats just plain look good, pause to consider how that choice will backfire on what you are trying to accomplish.

Data from the Third National Health and Nutrition Examination Survey have shown that Americans get 30% of their calories from junk food (nutrient-poor foods that are high in fat, sugar, or both). Only 10% of their caloric intake comes from fruit and vegetables. That's terrible!

This list, based on a 160-pound adult, estimates how much activity it would take to burn the calories from these goodies. If you weigh less, you burn fewer calories, and if you weigh more, you burn more calories.

100 Calories IN = 100 Calories OUT	
■ 4 Hershey's kisses	■ 2,000 steps
■ 2 mini-Reese's peanut butter cups	■ 8 minutes of jogging
■ 3 pieces of Bazooka gum	■ 10 minutes of
■ 1 small package of peanut M&Ms (0.7 ounce)	• basketball
	• chopping wood
■ Glass of wine (red or white)	• dancing (aerobic)
■ 1 light beer	• swimming at a moderate pace
■ 1 pale ale beer	■ 20 minutes of walking or
■ 4-ounce margarita	weightlifting
	■ 1 hour of bowling

(continued on page 178)

200 Calories IN = 200 Calories OUT

- 1 medium, plain croissant
- 4 Oreo cookies
- 18 Pringle's potato chips
- 1 KFC biscuit
- 1 slice of cheese or chicken pizza
- 1.8-ounce bag of Skittles
- 1 dark ale

- 4,000 steps
- 16 minutes of jogging
- 26 minutes of
  - skating (ice or rollerblade)
  - skiing (water or downhill)
  - tennis
  - shoveling snow
  - biking (about 10 mph)
- 30 minutes of
  - gardening
  - golfing (pull/carry clubs)
  - hiking
- 40 minutes of walking or weightlifting
- 70 minutes of golfing (power cart)

300 Calories IN = 300 Calories OUT

- 1 Snicker's candy bar (2.07 ounces)
- 1 old-fashioned cake donut
- 1 almond-filled croissant
- 5 Pepperidge Farm Milano cookies
- 1 McDonald's apple bran muffin (4 ounces)
- 1/2 cup premium ice cream

- 6,000 steps
- 24 minutes of jogging
- 30 minutes of
  - swimming
  - basketball
- 39 minutes of
  - skating (ice or rollerblade)
  - skiing (water or downhill)
  - tennis
  - shoveling snow
  - biking (about 10 mph)
- 45 minutes of gardening
- 60 minutes of walking or weightlifting
- 3 hours of bowling

400 Calories IN = 400 Calories OUT

- 1 Kit Kat bar (2.8 ounces)
- 1 brownie (3.5 ounces)
- 1 piece of tiramisu (5 ounces)
- 1 Green Tea Frappuccino (16 ounces)

- 8,000 steps
- 32 minutes of jogging
- 56 minutes of biking
- 64 minutes of golfing (pull/carry clubs) or hiking
- 1 hour, 50 minutes of social dancing
- 2 hours, 20 minutes of golfing (power cart)

Warning!

These examples were meant to clarify how quickly those calories from junk foods build up, not to justify eating junk food with a promise to "cancel it out" with exercise. It all counts. Consider this: According to Kevin D. Hall, PhD, of the National Institute of Diabetes and Digestive and Kidney Diseases, for the population to return to BMI values that prevailed in the 1970s, average diets would need to shrink by about 220 calories per day. That might seem like a lot, but it's easy to consume calorie-dense items if you are not conscious about it (just look at the pastry calories on your next trip to the local coffee shop).

I love my junk food: Are there any healthier options?

Here's a list of the top-five junk foods and alternative choices.

Junk	Healthier options	Why
Regular soda	Diet soda, water, sugar-free beverages, carbonated water, tea	Your body doesn't need the 8 teaspoons of sugar contained in a 12-ounce soda. Drinking water helps hydrate the body and keeps the kidneys happy.
Sweets, desserts, and pastries	Go with fruit instead or light or nonfat yogurt. Switch to dark chocolate in small amounts.	Fruit has no fat, few calories, and lots of fiber. Sweets are loaded with fat, sugar, and calories, which is the opposite of what you need. Dark chocolate has antioxidants and may benefit the blood vessels.
Fast food (hamburgers and fries)	Ask for your burger without cheese or mayonnaise. Try veggie burgers. Ask for a salad with low-fat dressing. Share the fries.	You can avoid lots of hidden calories, carbohydrates, and fat. And salt. And guilt. Get a fast-food nutrition guide or ask for a nutrition guide at your favorite fast-food places so you can identify healthier choices.
Pizza	Go for lower fat (vegetables) and fewer toppings. Share the pizza and avoid eating the whole thing in one sitting.	Pizza is the gift that keeps on giving. Pizza can raise blood glucose levels for hours and contains lots of fat and cholesterol.
Potato chips	Baked potato chips or a baked potato (not loaded with toppings). Try popcorn in place of chips.	Potato chips offer next to nothing in nutrients, except for fat, fat, and fat, plus some oil and salt. Baked potatoes are a healthy choice when topped only with veggies, baked beans, or cottage cheese.

PERSONAL GOAL

Date: _____ I will:

☐ Burn about 200 calories by walking to work or by walking during my break at work.

☐ Clear my cupboards of junk food and fill them with healthier options.

☐ Eat fast food only once a week.

☐ Order a calorie, fat gram, and carbohydrate counting book.

☐ Try an exercise I once enjoyed but haven't done in a while.

☐ Other:_____.

Sex burns 4 calories a minute.
Someone will be happy to hit that
"200 calories a day" mark.

WEEK
16

 Being Weigh Wise

Of the following tips to maintain weight, check the ones you are doing:

_____ Kept my eye on the prize (didn't forget my personal reason or motivator for this effort).

_____ Stayed accountable with a food and exercise diary (check out Day 8 for one to write on, or an online or smartphone app like The Eatery, myfitnesspal.com, or loseit.com).

_____ Practiced self-talk to help my thinking and thus behavior (e.g., "I can eat whatever I want, or I can be thinner").

_____ Used a hunger scale (1 = famished, 5 = starting to get hungry, 10 = stuffed) to help with the why, when, and how often I eat.

_____ Piled at least 1/3 of my plate with veggies.

_____ Ate breakfast every day this past week.

_____ Exercised for at least 30 minutes within the past 2 days.

_____ Recognized and dealt with my stress in a positive way.

Cholesterol Medications

Cholesterol building up in your blood vessels is like a smoldering fire. If ignored, it can overcome you when you least expect it. You can lower your cholesterol with your food choices and one of the following common cholesterol medications:

Types of cholesterol medicines	Brand name (generic name)	Possible side effects or issues
Statins* (work by reducing the liver's ability to make LDL cholesterol)	**Crestor** (rosuvastatin) **Lipitor** (atorvastatin) **Lescol** (fluvastatin) **Mevacor** (lovastatin) **Pravachol** (pravastatin) **Zocor** (simvastatin)	If you have muscle pain, notify your health-care provider immediately. Use caution when combined with fibric acid derivatives, bile acid sequestrants, or erythromycin because of a rare and potentially fatal condition called rhabdomyolysis. Usually taken at bedtime. Side effects can include insomnia, fatigue, depression, rash, and headaches. Not to be used during pregnancy.
Cholesterol Absorption Inhibitors (reduce total and LDL cholesterol levels by limiting absorption of cholesterol from food)	**Zetia** (ezetimibe)	Can be used alone or in combination with other drugs.
Fibric Acid Derivatives (reduce triglycerides and raise HDL cholesterol, but have little effect on LDL cholesterol)	**Atromid-S** (clofibrate) **Lopid** (gemfibrozil) **Tricor** (fenofibrate)	If you have muscle pain, notify your health-care provider immediately.

*Statin therapy is the preferred strategy to target LDL cholesterol and should be added to lifestyle therapy, regardless of baseline cholesterol (lipid) levels for people with diabetes.

Types of cholesterol medicines	Brand name (generic name)	Possible side effects or issues
Bile Acid Sequestrants (lower LDL cholesterol by binding to bile in the small intestine and preventing it from being absorbed into circulation)	**Colestid** (colestipol) **LoCholest** (cholestramine) **Questran** (cholestramine) **Prevalite** (cholestramine) **Welchol** (colesevelam)	May cause constipation and stomach upset. Taken once or twice a day with meals. Welchol may reduce blood glucose levels by 18 mg/dL after eating.
Nicotinic Acid (also known as niacin, increases HDL cholesterol levels, lowers LDL cholesterol, and lowers triglycerides)	**Niaspan and others** (nicotinic acid)	May increase insulin resistance and increase blood glucose levels. Frequent side effects include facial flushing and other skin conditions and worsening of gout or peptic ulcers. Take with food.
Combination	**Advicor** (lovastatin and niacin) **Juvisync** (sitagliptin and simvastatin) **Vytorin** (ezetimibe and simvastatin)	See descriptions above. Combination therapy has not been shown to provide additional cardiovascular benefit above statin therapy alone and generally is not recommended (per American Diabetes Association Standards of Care). For sitagliptin, see Day 12.

- ■ With existing CVD, a lower LDL goal of less than 70 mg/dL by using a higher dose of a statin is an option.
- ■ Without CVD but for people who are over the age of 40 years and have one or more other CVD risk factors (e.g., family history of CVD, hypertension, smoking, high cholesterol, or high levels of protein in the urine, called albuminuria).
- ■ Without CVD and younger than 40 years old if LDL remains more than 100 mg/dL or those with multiple CVD risk factors.

PERSONAL GOAL

Date: _____ I will:

☐ Eat low-fat choices.
☐ Call my health-care provider immediately if I am on one of these drugs and have muscle pain.
☐ Get copies of my recent liver function test and make sure I have one taken at least once a year.
☐ Take statins at bedtime.
☐ Take bile acid sequestrants with food.
☐ Report a flushed face, upset stomach, or constipation to my doctor.
☐ Other: _____.

 Mom gave me blue eyes, hammertoes, and high cholesterol. Dad gave me his love of fried foods. No wonder my pharmacist loves me.

WEEK
17

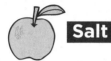

Salt

How about your salt intake?

Salt is ancient. Roman soldiers were believed to have been paid with salt, which was called a *salarium* in Latin. We call this a "salary." Now, fast forward to your table and consider these facts:

- According to the Food and Nutrition Board of the Institute of Medicine, an adequate intake of salt for adults ages 19–50 years is 1,500 milligrams, for ages 51–70 years it's 1,300 milligrams, and for ages 71 years and older it's 1,200 milligrams.
- 1 teaspoon of salt has 2,300 milligrams of sodium.
- The average daily sodium intake for Americans age 2 years and older is 3,436 milligrams.
- Some people are more sensitive to sodium than others, including people with hypertension, African Americans, and middle-age and older adults.
- More than 75% of dietary sodium comes from processed or packaged foods and from restaurant food.
- Decreasing sodium intake can decrease blood pressure. Adults in general should consume no more than 2,300 milligrams of sodium per day (or no more than 1,500 milligrams per day if you are 51 years of age or older, are African American, or have high blood pressure or chronic kidney disease). More than two out of every three people with diabetes also have high blood pressure.
- Increasing the amount of potassium in your diet can reduce the effects of sodium on blood pressure.

Season with spices instead

Discover the incredible flavors that spices have to offer. You may find that salt was a boring waste of time once you set foot into the rich world of herbs. Try some of these sumptuous alternatives and bring the exotic flavors of the world into your diet.

For meat, poultry, and tofu: allspice, basil, caraway seeds, cilantro, chives, curry powder, dill, dry mustard, garlic, ginger, lemon or lime juice, nutmeg, onion, paprika, turmeric, parsley, sage, rosemary, thyme

For fish: basil, curry powder, dill, garlic, lemon or lime juice, dry mustard, nutmeg, paprika, parsley, rosemary, sage, turmeric

For vegetables: cider vinegar, dill, garlic, dry mustard, dried oregano, lemon thyme, dried basil, onion, paprika, pimiento, rosemary, Italian seasoning, cilantro, sage

For salads: basil, caraway seeds, chives, cider/red wine or other flavored vinegar, cilantro, dried oregano, Italian seasoning, lemon or lime juice, onion, paprika, parsley, pimiento

For soups: basil, caraway seeds, chives, cilantro, curry powder, dried oregano, Italian seasoning, onion, paprika, parsley, cilantro

How to Shove That Salt Away

- Use fresh produce or frozen and canned items without added salt.
- Eat fresh fish, poultry, and lean meats instead of canned or smoked meats or cold cuts.
- Retire your saltshaker.
- Buy products that are salt free, sodium free, or low in sodium.
- Check the Nutrition Facts labels and choose brands that are lower in sodium.
- Read over-the-counter medication labels (some, like antacids and stool softeners, contain a lot of sodium).
- Go for cooked dry beans instead of canned beans.
- Pick unsalted nuts and seeds over the salted varieties.
- Consider using a salt substitute, but check with your doctor first. Potassium chloride salt substitutes are not safe for people with kidney problems.
- Eat lots of fruits and vegetables for potassium (the goal is at least 4,700 milligrams of potassium a day, but since many food labels don't list this information, it can be difficult to know whether you are getting enough potassium).

For fruit: allspice, almond extract, cinnamon, ginger, nutmeg, peppermint extract

For sauces: basil, chives, dill, dry mustard, paprika, parsley, rosemary, cilantro, turmeric

---

PERSONAL GOAL

Date: _____ I will:

☐ Taste my food before adding salt.

☐ Try a sodium-free dried spice during a meal rather than salt.

☐ Add up how much sodium I eat in a day.

☐ Choose low-sodium foods that contain no more than 140 milligrams of sodium per serving.

☐ Read labels to avoid added sodium (e.g., 4 ounces uncooked, skinless boneless Perdue chicken has 460 milligrams sodium compared to Tyson chicken, which has 160 milligrams).

☐ Ask my pharmacist about the sodium content of my prescription and over-the-counter medications (and for low-sodium alternatives). I won't stop my medication without my health-care provider's advice.

☐ Other: _____.

 Gone are the days of innocence . . . and salt.

MONTH 5

Laughin' Langerhans   By Theresa Garnero

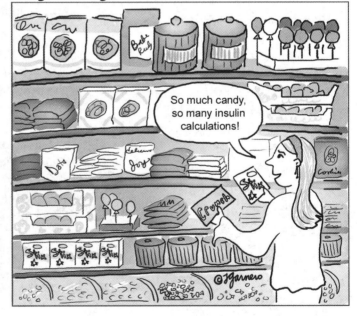

WEEK
18

Diabetes Isn't Sexy

Both men and women battle the issue of sex and diabetes. Although sex is so important to all of us, very few people are willing to discuss the complications that diabetes can bring into an otherwise healthy sex life.

"Don't ask, don't tell" in health care

Do you need proof that we aren't talking about sexual health in the health-care world? Fewer than 20% of people with diabetes who have sexual problems talk about it with their health-care providers. Worse yet, during regular medical visits, health-care providers rarely ask about sexual health.

Regardless of your sexual orientation, your health status, and your sexual life, you need to bring up sexual issues with your health-care providers if you have questions and he or she isn't asking you about them first. If you find that your health-care provider isn't willing to help you with your total health—including your sexual health—then it may be time to look around for a new health-care provider.

What Kinds of Sexual Problems Are Common in People with Diabetes?

- Lack of interest or decreased libido (more common in women than in men)
- Unable to climax (about the same frequency for women and men)
- Climax too quickly (more common in men than in women)
- Physical pain (more common in women than in men)
- Not pleasurable (more common in women than in men)
- Erection issues for men (at least one in four men)
- Lubrication issues for women (at least one in five women)

About 40% of men and women avoided sex because of these problems.

How Do You Avoid or Prevent Sexual Problems?

- **Prepregnancy planning.** An unplanned pregnancy adds unnecessary risks for your baby. If you want children, see an endocrinologist or obstetrician first to check which medications to stop and if switching to insulin will be necessary (certain diabetes pills, statins, and ACE inhibitors cause problems during pregnancy). It is important to maintain good blood glucose levels during pregnancy, too.
- **Glycemic control.** The better your blood glucose, the better your sex life. When blood glucose levels are in the target range, you'll have more energy to waltz down lover's lane.
- **Avoid hypoglycemia.** Sex is exercise (a *fun* type), and it can cause you to go low. Like any intense workout, you want to know what your blood glucose is before you start. You may need a preintimacy snack!
- **Limit alcohol.** Alcohol can lead to hypoglycemia. Making love in a state of hypoglycemia can turn a tender moment into a crisis.
- **Nutrition.** Those who eat better see a positive effect on sexual ability. Count those carbohydrates if you're using whipped cream or chocolate sauce. Semen and vaginal fluids do not have carbohydrates.
- **Exercise.** Those who exercise more have an increased ability in the bedroom.
- **Check hormones.** Low testosterone levels are more common in men than in women. This can cause loss of sex drive and depression. Replacement therapy is a possible treatment.
- **Don't be in a rush.** Making love should not be an environment in which you put yourself under pressure. Take your time. Roll out the red carpet. Play sexy music. Dim those lights and get flowers. Have a romantic dinner. Use foreplay. Be intimate with caresses. Use your imagination.
- **Communicate with your partner.** Unless you are with a mind reader, the only way your loved one will know what is going on is if you talk. Find out what pleases your partner, including experimenting with new positions, toys, or whatever rocks your world.

Special issues for men

Erectile dysfunction (ED) is the inability to get and maintain an erection and is the most common sexual problem for men. High levels of glucose can damage the nerves and blood vessels in the penis. When this happens, the interest in sex and the ability to perform it are two different things. Treatment for ED depends on your overall health status. Discuss treatment options with your health-care provider.

Treatments for ED

Following are treatments for ED:

- Pills (Cialis, Levitra, Viagra)
- Suppositories inserted into the tip of the penis (Muse)
- Pumps that bring blood into the penis
- Penile injections just before sex
- Implants

Note that other medications may cause ED (e.g., certain, but not all, blood pressure or depression pills).

Special issues for women

Uncontrolled diabetes can kill the mood for sexual relations and damage the nerves that affect vaginal lubrication. You may be interested in sex, but the dryness can cause pain. Over-the-counter personal lubricants can help. Menstrual cycles tend to send blood glucose levels higher, too. You may need more medications (for diabetes or pain), more exercise, or a slight reduction in carbohydrates in the diet. Conversely, during menopause, estrogen and progesterone levels drop, which contributes to dryness and may reduce the desire to have sex.

Other issues common to women with diabetes include vaginal yeast and urinary tract infections (UTIs). Yeast infections usually involve vaginal itching; a white, odorless "cheese-like" discharge; and pain with urination and sex. Yeast infections can be treated with over-the-counter medications. Also, eating low-fat yogurt with active cultures helps maintain the balance of healthy bacteria.

A UTI occurs when bacteria enters the bladder. Symptoms include a severe burning sensation during urination, the frequent urge to urinate (and only a few drops come out), foul-smelling urine, and pain on one side of your back. Left untreated, this can lead to a kidney infection and body-wide infection (sepsis). To treat a UTI, you will need an oral antibiotic from your health-care provider and to control blood glucose levels as much as possible (high glucose levels encourage bacteria to grow).

PERSONAL GOAL

Date: _____ I will:

☐ Tell my partner I am struggling with an issue related to sex.
☐ Ask to have my testosterone level tested and get copies of the results.
☐ Report sex-related concerns to my health-care provider.
☐ Take my time with sex.
☐ Buy an over-the-counter lubricant (K-Y jelly or Astroglide).
☐ Have a little snack before sex.
☐ Other: _____.

 I feel sorry for all the guys named ED.

Why do I need to check my blood pressure at home?

You can minimize your risk of future problems by knowing what your blood pressure is now and acting on those numbers. By checking at home, you'll have more information to work with than just an occasional check on your visits to your doctor.

What type of monitor is best?

For home use, select one with an inflatable cuff that goes over the arm or wrist. Highly rated home blood pressure monitors are made by Omron (www.omronhealthcare.com), microlife (www.microlifeusa.com), and Lifesource (www.andonline.com). Ask your pharmacist to point one out or order one for you.

When should I check my blood pressure?

Check your blood pressure regularly. Start off by checking first thing in the morning for a week. The next week, test at another time that is convenient, like after dinner. Definitely check your blood pressure if you feel any heart-related symptoms, such as skipped beats, shortness of breath, chest pain or pressure, dizziness, and nausea.

PERSONAL GOAL

Date: _____ I will:

☐ Buy a home blood pressure monitor.
☐ Check my blood pressure once a day or if I have chest pain, dizziness, sore neck or jaw, numbness in the arm, unexplained sweating, or nausea.
☐ Write down my readings and any comments about what I think might be influencing my readings (e.g., stress, late with medication, too much salt, too little exercise, too much exercise, etc.).
☐ Ask my health-care provider for instructions on when to call about my blood pressure.
☐ Bring my home blood pressure monitor to my next medical appointment to make sure my technique is correct.
☐ Bring my list of blood pressure readings to my next appointment and ask for a plan to improve my blood pressure.
☐ Other: _____.

My blood pressure monitor said, "Uh oh," all week.

Protein: From Beef to Beans to Barracuda

What is protein?

Protein is found in the meat and beans food group and contains materials needed to build up, maintain, and replace the body's cells. Cells are the smallest component of our bodies and the fundamental unit of living tissue, visible only under a microscope. Protein is necessary for the formation of hormones, enzymes, antibodies, muscles, skin, hair, nails, and internal organs.

How much protein do I need?

The recommended dietary allowance from protein is about 46 grams per day for women and 56 grams per day for men, although more or less may be needed based on weight, age, sex, and physical activity. Adults should get about 10–35% of their calories from protein.

It's pretty difficult to break down everything you eat into a percentage of calories, so take the easy way out: Follow the Plate Method (from Day 15) or try using the ounce equivalents as advised by the new food pyramid at choosemyplate.gov. Here's how it works: Count 1-ounce equivalents of protein to add up to the recommended 5-ounce equivalents for women or 6-ounce equivalents for men per day. Men are allowed more protein, so they'll have extra energy to take out the trash. Not really. It has to do with men having more muscle mass. Be sure to choose lean protein sources when adding up your 5- or 6-ounce equivalents.

Ounce-protein equivalent examples	Meat	Poultry	Seafood	Eggs/nuts	Beans/tofu
1	1 ounce lean beef	1 ounce skinless turkey or chicken (like a sandwich slice)	1 ounce cooked fish or shellfish	1 egg; 1 tablespoon peanut butter; 12 almonds; 24 pistachios; 2 tablespoons pumpkin or sunflower seeds	1/2 cup cooked beans (refried, black, white, pinto, kidney) or peas (lentils, split peas, chickpeas); 1/4 cup tofu; 1 falafel patty
2	2 ounces cooked pork or ham	2 ounces skinless turkey or chicken	1/2 can of drained tuna	4 tablespoons (1/4 cup) pumpkin or sunflower seeds; 3 egg whites	1 soy or tofu burger; 4 tablespoons hummus
3	1 small hamburger	1 small chicken breast	1 small trout	11 walnuts	1/4 cup wheat gluten
4	1 small steak (eye of round, filet)	1/2 Cornish game hen	1 salmon steak	This is left blank because it would be too many eggs or nuts for a serving size!	2 cups of lentil, or split pea, or bean soup

So, if you're a woman, you can have 4 tablespoons of sunflower seeds and a small chicken breast to meet your protein requirements for the day. A man can have 4 tablespoons of sunflower seeds and a small steak instead. Other combinations are possible, and this isn't even a complete list!

Does that look like too little food? Remember that we also get protein in our diets from other sources, including dairy products, starches, and some vegetables. These 5–6 ounces are based on the assumption that people will get extra protein from these other sources. In the U.S., we have no trouble getting enough protein: We consume almost twice the amount of protein—and fat for that matter—than is needed. Protein doesn't raise blood glucose like carbohydrates, but you need to be on the lookout for fat. Each gram of protein and carbohydrate contains 4 calories, but fat contains 9 calories per gram. Those calories can add up quickly.

What is considered a lean source of protein?

Get yourself lean and mean by choosing protein sources that are baked, broiled, barbequed (while holding off on the BBQ sauce), steamed, or grilled but not fried. For all meats, trim off excess fat and remove skin from poultry. Here are examples of lean protein:

- Beef round
- Fresh pork or ham
- Sirloin
- Skinless chicken or turkey breast
- Tofu or wheat gluten

What about fish?

The omega-3 fat content of fish has been shown to help protect against coronary artery disease. Generally, the darker the meat on a fish (like salmon, herring, and mackerel), the more omega-3 fatty acids it has. Conversely, the lighter the meat (such as cod and flounder), the less omega-3 it'll have. Some fish, like trout and salmon, contain more fat than some beef choices. To make a healthy fish choice, just avoid eating it fried. Fried calamari may taste yummy, but can your arteries afford that luxury?

An Argument for a Vegetarian Diet

Vegetarians are herbivores. They do not eat animal flesh. Ovo-lacto vegetarians include dairy products, such as eggs, cheese, and milk, in their diets, whereas vegans do not eat (and often don't wear or use) anything of animal origin. Research suggests that vegetarianism makes for good health. The cornerstone of a vegetarian diet is vegetables.

Those who eat meat have *three* times the obesity rate of vegetarians and *nine* times the obesity rate of vegans. Vegetarians have the lowest rate of coronary artery disease of any group with a fraction of the heart attack rate and 40% less cancer than those who eat meat (except for South Asians, although their risk is lowered when they follow a vegetarian diet). Plus, on average, vegetarians and vegans live 6–10 years longer than meat eaters. The downside? The longer you live, the more taxes you'll pay.

Many people are concerned that following a vegetarian diet means that it will be tough to get enough protein or calcium. This is true for people who do not carefully put together their meal plans, but vitamin and mineral supplements can be used to ensure that you get the proper nutrients. In general, though, following a healthy vegetarian diet will provide enough protein and calcium, which can be found in tofu products, whole-wheat bread, oatmeal, beans, legumes, nuts, and broccoli. If you eat a variety of unrefined grains, legumes, seeds, nuts, and vegetables throughout the day, even if one food is low in a particular essential nutrient, another food will make up this deficit. There are tons of vegetarian options out there, including tofu, wheat gluten, tempeh, mycoprotein (seen in the product with the brand name of Quorn), textured vegetable protein, egg replacers, and nondairy "dairy" products. Try a few; you may be surprised by how much you like them.

What about a Vegan Diet?

A vegan diet is a diet in which no animal products are consumed. That means not only avoiding meat and fish, as in a vegetarian diet, but also foods made from animals, such as dairy products, honey, and eggs. At this point, you may be racking your brain to think, what's left for me to eat? In fact, you still have plenty of options and can lead a healthy lifestyle with diabetes as a vegan. Here are some ideas to consider:

Comparing Animal to Vegetable Meal Options

Out with the animal (old meal)	In with the vegetable (new meal)
Breakfast: ■ Sausage links, scrambled eggs, and toast with butter ■ Cereal with milk and a blueberry muffin	**Breakfast:** ■ Gimme Lean fat-free "sausage," tofu scrambler, and toast with jam ■ Cereal with soy milk or oatmeal with cinnamon and raisins and a banana
Lunch: ■ Grilled cheese sandwich and creamy tomato soup ■ Chicken and cheese quesadilla, tortilla chips with sour cream and salsa	**Lunch:** ■ Lettuce, tomato, and hummus sandwich and split-pea soup ■ Black bean and sweet-potato burrito with corn and tomatoes and tortilla chips with salsa
Dinner: ■ Beef stir-fry and white rice ■ Spaghetti and meatballs with marinara sauce and parmesan cheese	**Dinner:** ■ Vegetable stir-fry seasoned with low-sodium soy sauce served over brown rice ■ Vegetable lasagna with low-fat tofu instead of ricotta, layered with grilled vegetables

For desserts, try tasty fresh fruit, smoothies, or dairy-free sorbet. Snacks can include baby carrots dipped in hummus, air-popped popcorn, or baked tortilla chips with salsa.

PERSONAL GOAL

Date: _____ I will:

☐ Try out one of the vegan meals in the meal table.
☐ Barbeque some cubed fruit at a cookout.
☐ Check out a local vegan restaurant with a friend.
☐ Plant some tomatoes in my back yard.
☐ Bake an apple or pear for dessert.
☐ Keep blueberries in the freezer for a snack.
☐ Support those soybean farmers: Try tofu!
☐ Visit www.choosemyplate.gov for an inside look at protein requirements.
☐ Try an egg substitute.
☐ Other: _____.

Albert Einstein was a vegetarian who found the relativity of wheat gluten as a hair product.

Insulin Is In

At least 30% of people with type 2 diabetes need insulin. The hormone insulin is life sustaining—we need it like we need air. If your body is not making enough insulin, you have to get it somehow. Insulin is the most powerful tool out there for managing diabetes.

One of the most common hurdles to starting insulin therapy is the fear of needles. This is understandable, but technology has vastly improved methods of insulin delivery with much smaller, shorter needles and needle-less systems. There are a lot of myths surrounding insulin. Insulin doesn't cause complications; having long periods of high blood glucose levels does. A CDE or a member of your health-care team can help you learn how to take insulin.

If I need insulin, does that mean my diabetes is really bad?

No, it does not. It just means that your pancreas is not producing as much insulin anymore, and injecting insulin will help you in your diabetes self-care.

What are the types of insulin?

Insulin falls into two broad categories:
- *Rapid or short-acting insulin (mealtime or correction)*—covers your meals or corrects a high blood glucose reading.
- *Long-acting insulin (background or basal)*—provides a steady level of insulin throughout the day and night.

How much insulin do I need?

On the basis of your glucose patterns, your health-care provider will decide the type of insulin approach to take.

What is insulin action?

Think of insulin action like popping popcorn. The kernels of corn don't pop all at once. A few kernels pop first, then most pop at once, and a few leftover kernels pop at the end. Similarly, insulin doesn't all work at once. There is a delay; then it starts to kick in (known as *onset*), most of it works at its strongest for a certain amount of time (known as the *peak*), and some of it lingers in your system, but does not have as strong an effect (known as the *duration*). Many new types of insulin are under investigation and may be available by the time you read this.

Insulin type	Brand name (generic name)	Onset	Peak	Duration	Notes
Mealtime or correction Rapid-acting	**Apidra** (glulisine)	5–10 minutes	1–2 hours	3–4 hours	If using with a meal, make sure you do not delay the meal. If you are eating out, don't inject until your meal has been delivered. If you skip a meal, skip this, too, unless you are taking a dose to correct a high glucose level as advised by your provider.
	Humalog (lispro)				
	NovoLog (aspart)				
Short-acting	**Humulin R** or **Novolin R** (regular)	30 minutes	2–4 hours	4–8 hours	
Background or basal Intermediate-acting	**Humulin N Novolin N** (NPH), ReliOn	2–4 hours	6–10 hours	Up to 20 hours	Be sure to roll (do not shake) the vial or pen to mix the solution before injecting.
Long-acting	**Lantus** (glargine)	1–2 hours	Peak-less	Up to 24 hours	Avoid mixing with other insulins in the same syringe. Take about the same time daily. Don't skip doses.
	Levemir (detemir)				
Combination or premixed insulin 70/30	Humulin 70% NPH/ 30% regular ReliOn; Novolin 70% NPH/ 30% regular NovoLog Mix; 70% insulin aspart/ 30% insulin aspart protamine	10–30 minutes	2–12 hours	Up to 24 hours	Roll the vial or rotate the pen several times before use.
75/25	75% NPH/ 25% lispro	Less than 15 minutes	3–12 hours	Up to 24 hours	Roll the vial or rotate the pen several times before use.
50/50	Humulin 50% NPH/ 50% regular	Less than 30 minutes	4–8 hours	Up to 24 hours	Roll the vial or rotate the pen several times before use.
U-500 Regular	Humulin R U-500	30 minutes	2–4 hours	Up to 24 hours	See page 205.

Let's stay cool: insulin storage

Bottles (vials). Keep unopened vials of insulin in the refrigerator (36–46°F) and opened ones at room temperature (59–86°F; for glulisine: less than 77°F). Insulin is easier to inject (i.e., less burning sensation) when it is at room temperature. Once a vial has been opened (whether or not it is in the fridge), it is only good for 28 days (except detemir, which can be kept at room temperature for 42 days). This means you need to throw away unused insulin after the vial has been opened for this amount of time, regardless of whether the expiration date on the bottle has passed.

Pens. Keep insulin pens at room temperature. Expiration dates vary among different pen manufacturers, so check the package inserts or ask your pharmacist. Generally, 75/25 insulin expires 10 days after opening; 70/30 expires in 14 days; glulisine, lispro, aspart, and regular insulin expire in 28 days; and detemir expires in 42 days.

Where can I inject the insulin?

Insulin should be injected into the abdomen (stomach area), upper or outer arms, outer thighs, and buttocks in the subcutaneous or fat area just below the skin. Don't inject near scars and stay at least 2 inches away from your belly button. Rotate your injection sites to avoid developing scar tissue.

What sites absorb insulin the quickest?

Insulin is absorbed the fastest from the following sites in the following order (from fastest to slowest): abdomen, arms, legs, and buttocks. If you tend to have lower blood glucose levels, you might consider injecting into a site that absorbs more slowly, like the buttocks or thigh. Conversely, if you tend to have higher blood glucose levels, you might want to inject into your abdomen, which will absorb it more quickly and more consistently than other sites.

Needles and sharps disposal

If you use needles and syringes, check into your local regulations; call your waste management company to find out what options are

If You Need It: U-500

Some people are highly resistant to insulin and require more than 200 units a day. If this applies to you, then regular U-500 insulin (which has five times the strength of the standard U-100 insulin concentration) may be prescribed. U-500 insulin has an onset similar to regular insulin, peaks in 2–4 hours, and may last as long as 24 hours. It's usually taken in two to three injections using a different type of syringe that has volume, instead of unit, markings (called a tuberculin syringe). Alternatively, your provider may have you use regular U-100 insulin syringes and convert the numbers because tuberculin syringes can be hard to find. Pre-dinner doses are usually smaller than pre-breakfast doses to minimize the risk of nighttime hypoglycemia. If you need U-500, you need to see a CDE. It is the only insulin sold in 20-milliliter vials. The labels on the box and bottle have a red label, "Warning—High Potency Not for Ordinary Use."

Other Insulin Tips

- Don't ever use insulin that is or has been frozen. Throw it out.
- Sometimes insulin leaks out a little after being injected. If this happens to you, count to five before withdrawing the needle.
- If you have a tendency to bruise, make sure that you are not injecting too fast, that your insulin is at room temperature, that you have a short needle, and that you are rotating injection sites.
- Wash your hands before injecting! Alcohol is generally not needed to wipe the skin unless it is dirty or covered with lotion.
- Keep a back-up supply of insulin so you never run out.
- Insert the needle straight in at a 90-degree angle. (Needle size is covered in Month 6, Week 22.)
- If you are mixing insulin in one syringe (but never glargine or detemir), start with the clear one and go to cloudy. If you miscalculate, throw it away and start over.
- Where there is air in the syringe, there is no insulin. A little air won't hurt you, but it does mean you are not getting the full dose of insulin. If you see an air bubble, either tap it out or, if you are dealing with one type of insulin, push it rapidly back into the vial and the bubble should go away.
- Adjust insulin doses under the guidance of your health-care provider. See Month 6, Week 22 for some general guidelines.

near you. Your community may have a sharps container pick-up service or drop-off center (some pharmacies offer this as well). Not all municipalities require special disposal. Needles and lancets should not be tossed away in the trash like the rest of your garbage because they might poke someone who handles the trash. If you are allowed to dispose of sharps in the trash, use a puncture-resistant container and seal the lid securely. There are also some national mail-back services that are either independent (check your local pharmacy) or associated with a syringe and needle manufacturer, such as BD (www.bd.com/sharps).

Glucagon: Overdraft Protection against Severe Lows

Glucagon is a hormone naturally produced by the alpha-cells in the pancreas. When glucose is low, glucagon is released and tells the liver to release glucose.

If you are on insulin and have ever had a severe low blood glucose level where you passed out or were not fully awake to treat the situation personally (which may occur when glucose levels fall below 50 mg/dL—but everyone has their own threshold as to how "low" they can tolerate), you should have a glucagon injection kit and show your family or friends how to use it. When glucagon is injected, it quickly raises blood glucose levels to bring you out of unconsciousness. It's common to feel nauseated or to vomit immediately after awakening from a glucagon injection. Because the rise in glucose caused by glucagon is short lived, you must immediately ingest some form of carbohydrate, such as glucose gel or juice.

PERSONAL GOAL

Date: _____ I will:

☐ Not take rapid- or short-acting insulin until I am ready to eat.
☐ Take my glargine or detemir about the same time every day.
☐ On my calendar, mark the expiration dates for insulin vials or pens after I open them.
☐ Keep unopened insulin vials in the refrigerator and opened ones at room temperature.
☐ Go out for a walk to improve the way my body uses insulin.
☐ Call my local waste management company to find out about local needle disposal regulations.
☐ Start a new vial of insulin if I suddenly see an increase in my blood glucose levels.
☐ Ask my doctor about new insulins.
☐ Other: _____.

I'm insulin resistant.
I'm resistant to taking insulin.

WEEK
21

 Your Virtual Community

Imagine a support group that could meet on *your* terms, when it is convenient, even in your home in that odd 45 minutes of spare time you have at 10 p.m. The diabetes online community (DOC) can do just that, virtually. The DOC includes websites, blogs, online forums, Facebook pages, and Twitter handles that connect you with people with diabetes from all walks of life, all over the world. You can communicate with others in similar situations, find support, and learn about new diabetes technologies or great insider tips for staying motivated to care for yourself.

Although it would be ideal for everyone to have an in-person diabetes support network, this isn't always feasible. Maybe you feel like your friends or spouse don't "get it" when it comes to your diabetes. Maybe you have tangible support but could use some more. Following are some reliable sources through which you can meet the DOC:

American Diabetes Association (ADA)
www.diabetes.org
1-800-DIABETES (342-2383)
For the official, science-backed standard of care, start your search engine here! Learn how best to manage diabetes, find new developments, and access plenty of resources. *Diabetes Forecast* is the stellar Association magazine for members. The ADA is also the publisher of this lovely book.

American Association of Diabetes Educators
www.diabeteseducator.org
1-800-338-3633
The professional association dedicated to ensuring the delivery of high-quality diabetes education. Locate the nearest diabetes educator by clicking on the "Find a Diabetes Educator" icon on the home page.

Academy of Nutrition and Dietetics

www.eatright.org

Provides multiple nutrition and health resources and a way to find an RD.

Choose My Plate

www.choosemyplate.gov

Build your plate with foods that are right for you. Wealth of info, tip of the day, SuperTracker, and weight management resources.

Diabetes Daily

www.diabetesdaily.com

Offers popular topics in the community, diabetes news and headlines on the web, and many online community groups.

Diabetes Health Magazine

www.DiabetesHealth.com

1-415-883-1990

A monthly magazine that focuses on living well with diabetes, including product reviews and diabetes cartoons.

Diabetes Health Monitor

www.healthmonitor.com/diabetes

A comprehensive website with a free magazine that is distributed six times a year.

Diabetes Mine

www.diabetesmine.com

A gold mine of straight talk and encouragement. Also has diabetes cartoons.

dLife

www.dlife.com

Offers expert columns, inspiration, food database, cooking videos, and multiple online support groups. Previous cable episodes and current shows all online.

Insulin Independence

www.insulindependence.org

1-888-912-3837

Inspires people with diabetes to set personal fitness goals and explore individual capacities. (The former Diabetes Exercise and Sports Association merged here.)

Joslin Diabetes Center
www.joslin.org
1-617-309-2400
An internationally known institution devoted to the study and treatment of diabetes.

JDRF
www.jdrf.org
1-800-533-2873
Focuses on type 1 diabetes, especially in children, as well as activities, research, advocacy, and publications.

MedicAlert
www.medicalert.org
1-888-633-4298
Helps get critical health information to providers in an emergency situation 24 hours a day anywhere in the world. Offers customized medical bracelets and necklaces.

Mendosa.com
www.mendosa.com
A freelance medical writer with diabetes, specializing in diabetes. Get the inside scoop here.

National Diabetes Education Program (NDEP)
ndep.nih.gov
1-301-496-3583
NDEP is a partnership of the National Institutes of Health, the Centers for Disease Control and Prevention, and more than 200 public and private organizations. Check out their new Diabetes HealthSense site, which gives you tools to live well and meet your goals. Includes videos on behavior change and multicultural materials.

National Diabetes Information Clearinghouse
www.diabetes.niddk.nih.gov
1-800-860-8747
An information service of the National Institute of Diabetes and Digestive and Kidney Diseases, part of the National Institutes of Health that covers diabetes, care, treatment, and medical resources.

National Institutes of Health
www.nlm.nih.gov/medlineplus/diabetes.html
www.Medlineplus.com (click on "diabetes")
Provides a robust library (including videos and in multiple languages) of understandable medical information for people with diabetes.

PERSONAL GOAL

Date: _____ I will:

☐ Visit at least one of the websites mentioned in this section.

☐ Find a way to access the Internet (e.g., public libraries, ask a younger relative, a neighbor).

☐ Send a message online to one person I come across through the DOC.

☐ Watch an online video about diabetes.

☐ Visit www.twitter.com and put "diabetes" in the search box.

☐ Subscribe to a free or paid diabetes journal, or call any diabetes journal and ask if they have a free issue for me to preview.

☐ Ask my pharmacist or CDE for a free diabetes magazine.

☐ Other: _____.

 "What's up, DOC?" has a whole new meaning.

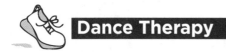
Dance Therapy

The fun type of exercise

Life, like diabetes, is a dance: full of complex rhythms, melodies, and of course discord, but there is a way to have fun while being healthy. Dancing often is described as a source of joy. Just look at the smiles on the dance floor.

Even if you don't consider yourself a dancer, moving your body to music you enjoy has many benefits, including the following:

- Improves balance, endurance, strength, flexibility, and memory.
- Enhances sense of well-being, social ties, and diabetes management.
- Offers a fun way to burn calories and maintain weight.

One study showed that dancing twice a week for just 12 weeks produced significant improvements in blood pressure, body fat, and A1C (not to mention the enjoyment, laughter, and camaraderie experienced on the dance floor).

Think about how we typically gain 3 pounds every winter. As we age, we lose muscle mass and tend to exercise less, and as a result, insulin resistance follows. You can slow down this process by regular physical activity. The trick is finding something you *enjoy*. Could it be dance and you don't know it yet?

You can dance just about anywhere, starting in your living room, or for a 1-minute break at work when no one is looking. Put on your favorite music and let yourself move. Given the many types of dance genres, you may want to try out a few to find the one you prefer.

PERSONAL GOAL

Date: _____ I will:

☐ Do a little dance today.
☐ Check out a local dance class (like Zumba, hip-hop, line dancing).
☐ Visit www.danceoutdiabetes.org for online options and safety tips.
☐ Ask a buddy to go dancing.
☐ Bail on the dance idea and check out www. letsmove.gov to inspire other options.
☐ Other: _____.

Would you risk striking a pose to improve your health? Say yes!

MONTH 6

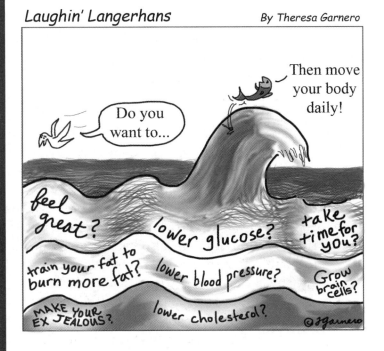

Laughin' Langerhans — By Theresa Garnero

Finding Insulin Harmony

This week will focus on insulin delivery and strategies used to fine-tune insulin dosage. This overview is not intended to replace the individualized care you need to receive from your health-care provider. But you can use this information as a starting point to discuss options with whoever prescribed your insulin.

Delivery options

We have come a long way from glass syringes with hand-sharpened needles and injections of thick, brown solutions made from ground-up cow pancreases that required injecting well over 20 times the amount of insulin than is used today. Technology now offers people with diabetes many insulin-delivery systems.

Syringe and vial. This was the first insulin-delivery system available and is the most common way to take insulin. It is usually the most economical, too. You manually draw up the insulin and inject it yourself.

Insulin pens. This is a popular, easy-to-use option with self-contained insulin in the shape of a small pen. Insulin pens offer a convenient way to carry and discreetly use insulin in public. Be sure to "prime" the pen (also known as an "air shot") by discarding 2 units into the trash. This makes sure you will get the full dose by eliminating any spaces of air in the system. Also, after the needle is inserted, push down *firmly* on the plunger for 3–5 seconds to be certain you get the full amount. Do not store the pen with the pen needle attached, and replace the needle after each use. Some systems include a clicking sound to indicate the number of units dialed up, which makes them suitable for people with vision problems. *Warning to left-handed people:* Be careful to read the units correctly. You accidentally could take 9 units instead of 6 units with some systems because the numbers will be reversed when using your left hand.

Insulin pumps. Pumps continuously deliver insulin through a device about the size of a pager and a tiny, plastic tube inserted under the skin. It has revolutionized the way in which diabetes is managed. The benefits include fewer injections (because you only change the plastic tube, or catheter tubing, every 3 days) and improved freedom from rigid schedules. The disadvantages are the initial intensive training required to properly use the device and the necessity to check glucose levels 6–10 times a day.

What is the best syringe?

The answer to this question is different for every individual, but three components to making your decision are syringe size, needle length, and needle width.

Syringe size. The syringe size is based on the "cc" mark (or cubic centimeter) that indicates the volume of insulin in the syringe when filled to that marker. The three basic syringe sizes are 1 cc (holds up to 100 units), 1/2 cc (holds up to 50 units), and 3/10 cc (holds up to 30 units). Make sure your syringe can hold slightly more than the amount of insulin you are taking; this makes it easy to see how much insulin you are getting. Most syringes have 1-unit measurements. A few brands offer 1/2-unit or 2-unit measurements.

Needle length. You'll also need a needle length that's suitable to your body type. Needles are available in 4 millimeters (5/32 inch), 5 millimeters (3/16 inch), 8 millimeters (5/16 inch), and 12.7 millimeters (1/2 inch) lengths. The 4-millimeter pen needle length allows for a straight-in, no-pinch injection technique.

Needle width. Manufacturers offer several gauges (needle width or thickness) to provide a more comfortable injection. You can find needle gauges of 28, 29, 30, 31, and 32 (the higher the gauge number, the thinner the needle thickness).

Can I reuse my insulin syringes?

Can you or should you? It's generally best to never reuse a syringe.

The needles are so fine that, on a microscopic level, the needle tip bends with reuse and causes tissue damage and pain. The other risk is that you can contaminate your insulin bottle by not using a sterile needle (*never* clean *any* needle or lancet with an alcohol wipe, as this will only introduce bacteria and might remove the protective coating intended to reduce pain). If you mix two types of insulin, reusing the syringe will contaminate your insulin bottles. And never reuse an insulin pen needle because the device may not function properly and you might dose incorrectly.

How to Adjust Insulin

Warning: When adjusting insulin, please work with your health-care provider. Although the following suggestions may be common approaches to insulin dose adjustment, you want to ensure that you are safe and under the guidance of a professional before changing your insulin program. It takes time to understand these steps and to see how your body responds.
Suggestion: Review each step carefully. This is intense!

1. **Be consistent and patient.** If you make an insulin dose adjustment, change *one* insulin dose by a small amount and keep the dosage consistent. This is the only way to see the effect on overall patterns.
2. **Fix the fasting first.** If your glucose values jump around like a hyperactive kid on a pogostick, it helps to focus on the first value of the day. Basal, or background, insulin has the most effect on the fasting glucose. Once the fasting value is in the target range of 70–130 mg/dL, the rest of the glucose values are more likely to follow suit. Adjust the long-acting insulin (Lantus, Levemir, NPH) by 1 unit every day until the fasting is at target. If you are awakened by a low glucose (less than 70), have nightmares, or soak the bed with sweat, lower the next insulin dose by at least 2 units, and notify your health-care provider.

    Note: It is important to maintain a balance between the amount of units you take per day for background insulin (roughly 50% of your total daily dose) and the units you take per day of mealtime or correction insulin (roughly 50%). These percentages are an estimated starting place. You and your health-care provider will find the right percentage of background to mealtime and correction insulin for your situation.

3. **Figure out your insulin-to-carbohydrate ratio.** For those taking rapid-acting insulin before meals (Humalog, NovoLog, Apidra), you can learn how many grams of carbohydrates 1 unit of insulin covers. (Do not attempt this until your basal insulin has been calculated to give you a pattern of fairly stable, in-range fasting glucose values; otherwise, you can miscalculate the insulin-to-carb ratio and need to make further mealtime or bolus adjustments.) [*Source*: "Tune in to Your Ratio(s)," by Gary Scheiner, MS, CDE, in *Diabetes Self-Management* (March/April 2006).]

   Gather 2 weeks' worth of glucose data. Check your glucose before one meal and 3 hours later, and try not to exercise, snack, or take extra insulin during that time, to eliminate variables. Ideally, your glucose pre- and postmeal should be within 30 points for this purpose. Start with breakfast and note whether the insulin-to-carb ratio made your glucose increase, stay the same, or drop. For example, let's look at 1 week's worth of data:

Date	Prebreakfast glucose	Grams of carb eaten	Units of rapid-acting insulin	Insulin-to-carb ratio (carb divided by units of insulin)	3 hours post-breakfast glucose	Comments
2/1	151	42	6	1:7[a]	93	1:7 ratio makes glucose drop
2/2	123	50	5	1:10[b]	86	1:10 makes glucose drop a little
2/3	295	20	7	1:3[c]	65	1:3 makes glucose drop a lot
2/4	83	50	4	1:12[d]	78	1:12 held glucose about the same
2/5	75	75	5	1:15[e]	180	1:15 makes glucose rise
2/6	168	60	5	1:12[f]	171	1:12 held glucose about the same
2/7	62	75	5	Don't use	226	Don't count due to hypoglycemia

a. 42 carbohydrates divided by 6 units = 7 points of glucose affected by 1 unit of insulin.
b. 50 carbohydrates divided by 5 units = 10 points of glucose affected by 1 unit of insulin.
c. 20 carbohydrates divided by 7 units = 3 points of glucose affected by 1 unit of insulin.
d. 50 carbohydrates divided by 4 units = 12 points of glucose affected by 1 unit of insulin.
e. 75 carbohydrates divided by 5 units = 15 points of glucose affected by 1 unit of insulin.
f. 60 carbohydrates divided by 5 units = 12 points of glucose affected by 1 unit of insulin.

In this chart, you can see that the 1:12 insulin-to-carbohydrate ratio held the glucose steady. You'd need another week's worth of data to determine whether 1:12 had the best track record for you. Also note any such variables as work, stress, exercise, infections, dining out, and so on.

Copy this form to determine your insulin-to-carb ratios for breakfast, lunch, and dinner. Here is where the patience part comes in. This may take you a good 6 weeks to figure out. Remember to discard data from the days that have unusual extremes (illness, hypoglycemic episodes, etc.), as you are looking for patterns of stable conditions with which to determine insulin-to-carb ratios.

Date	Prebreakfast glucose	Grams of carb eaten	Units of rapid-acting insulin	Insulin-to-carb ratio (carb divided by units of insulin)	3 hours post-breakfast glucose	Comments

MEAL (pick one to focus on for up to 2 weeks) _____

MY IDEAL INSULIN-TO-CARB RATIO _____

Insulin-to-carb ratios vary during different times of the day. It's not uncommon to have lower insulin-to-carb ratios in the morning and higher ratios for lunch and dinner. This can mean you start out with a 1:12 for breakfast, move up to a 1:14

for lunch, and reach a 1:17 for dinner. It's all based on your patterns, trial and error, and consideration of how variables affect your insulin requirements (like exercise, needing more insulin before menstruation, stress, amount of sleep, pain, etc.).

4. **Correct high premeal values or the "correction factor."** Once your fasting is in target more times than not, and you have figured out your carb-to-insulin ratio to cover your meal, you are ready for more fine-tuning: correcting high, premeal glucose values or the "correction factor." This also is known as the "insulin sensitivity factor" because your response (or sensitivity) to insulin can and often does change over time. This is not to bog you down with details, but rather to help you to be aware of the terms used.

    Follow the 1,800 rule. The 1,800 rule lets you set up a personal scale to *correct* high glucose values. Add up your total daily dose of all units of insulin and divide into 1,800. [Alternatively: To estimate how much 1 unit of rapid-acting insulin (NovoLog, Humalog, Apidra) will drop your glucose, take 1,800 and divide by the total daily dose of all insulin.]

    A common correction factor is 1 unit of rapid-acting insulin (NovoLog, Humalog, Apidra) to lower 50 mg/dL of glucose.

    Note: The correction bolus can be used only after your basal or background rates are set to prevent lows.

Take 1,800 and divide by your total daily insulin dose	To calculate the points of glucose drop per 1 unit of rapid-acting insulin
20 units	90
25 units	75
30 units	60
35 units	51
40 units	45
50 units	36
60 units	30
75 units	24
100 units	18

1,800 divided by _____ (TOTAL daily insulin) = _____ points glucose drop per 1 unit.

In the previous chart, for someone taking 35 units total insulin units a day, 1 unit of rapid-acting insulin would be expected to lower glucose by 51 points. This correction factor would be written as 1:51, which means 1 unit of rapid-acting insulin would be expected to drop glucose 51 mg/dL.

"Correct" your target glucose. To correct your target glucose, you first need to know what your target (or goal) is for your baseline glucose. Let's practice. Let's say your glucose target before meals is 100 mg/dL, and your current reading is 253 mg/dL. You would subtract 100 from 253, which equals 153 (points that need "correcting" to get you to your goal glucose of 100). Based on the previous example of a correction factor of 51, divide 153 by 51 and you get 3. It would take 3 units of rapid-acting insulin to correct your glucose to the baseline of 100.

Note: If you are taking regular insulin, use the 1,500 rule (take 1,500 divided by your total daily dose to calculate how many points of glucose will drop per 1 unit of regular insulin). The 1,500 Rule for Regular was developed by Dr. Paul Davidson and was modified to the rule of 1,800 for faster-acting insulins.

5. **Add the units of insulin-to-carb ratio dose with the units from your premeal correction factor dose.** One way to conceptualize this is to think of correction factor as correcting the past (high glucose). Your insulin-to-carb ratio or mealtime insulin predicts your best guess at covering the future (glucose levels) in response to your food. Put them together in one injection.

   Once you know how to correct for a high glucose, you can add that number to your insulin-sensitivity factor to project coverage for what you are about to eat.

   In other words, take your insulin-to-carb dose _____ units and add in your correction dose _____ units, to equal your premeal dose _____. It takes practice and guidance from your health-care team.

6. **Factor in exercise.** On the days you exercise, you may need to lower your basal or background dose by 2 to 4 units or more, depending on the type and intensity of exercise.

7. **Plan for illness.** Insulin requirements during illness actually can increase. Work with your health-care provider to come up with a plan ahead of time, before you get sick.

8. **Handle missed insulin doses.**
   a. **Once-a-day, intermediate, or long-acting insulin.**
      If you missed your once-a-day, intermediate, or long-acting insulin dose, and you realize it within 4 hours, the full dose can be taken. If it's more than 4 hours late, calculate the number of hours late, divide by 24, and multiply by your usual insulin dose.
   b. **Twice-a-day, intermediate, or long-acting insulin.** If you missed your twice-a-day, intermediate, or long-acting insulin dose, and it's within 4 hours, you can take the full dose. If it's more than 4 hours, skip that dose entirely and cover any high glucose levels with rapid-acting insulin.
   c. **Mealtime dose of rapid-acting insulin.** If you missed a mealtime dose of rapid-acting insulin and realize it within the hour, take your normal dose. If it's within 2 hours late, take 75% of your normal dose, and if it's 3 hours late, take 50% of your normal dose. If you use a personalized scale, you can recheck your glucose and use a correction factor instead. (*Source:* Adapted from *JoslinEZstart Resource Manual*, 2006.)

9. **Adjust insulin when traveling.** Are you traveling East and losing more than 3–4 hours of your 24-hour day? If you are on Lantus or Levemir, you can continue to take it at the same time as your "old" time zone. If you take an intermediate-acting insulin (NPH), reduce the amount equal to the percentage of day lost (if you lost 6 hours, that equals 25%, which would equal a 25% reduction in NPH dose). Your other option is to skip the NPH dose and cover with rapid-acting insulin every 3–4 hours until you arrive, in which case you can resume NPH on the "new" time zone at the time you normally would take it at home.

   If you are going west and gaining 3–4 hours and using Lantus or Levemir, you can continue to take it at the same time or gradually adjust by 1–2 hours each day until it is adjusted back to your home time after you return. If you are on NPH, you may need extra rapid-acting insulin with meals.

   Note: if you run out of insulin and are in some European or Latin American countries, they may use Insulin U-40, so best to use U-40 syringes. Ask for help on this. (*Source:* Adapted from *JoslinEZstart Resource Manual,* 2006.)

10. **Use more than just a calculator.** Calculating insulin doses based on the historical data that led up to the point the glucose value was measured, while projecting future glucose trends and the necessary insulin coverage, requires thought and perseverance. Sometimes glucose patterns have no rhyme or reason, which can be a huge source of frustration. Don't go it alone.

This is a case of the more you know, the more you realize you don't know. Insulin does a body great. Insulin adjustment is somewhat of a fine art. With guidelines, support, and practice, you can have an insulin plan that more closely mimics the work of the pancreas.

PERSONAL GOAL

Date: _____ I will:

☐ Go step-by-step with this guide and work with my health-care provider to get the best insulin dose to manage my diabetes.

☐ Have my health-care provider double check my insulin-delivery technique.

☐ Ask about the Freestyle InsuLinx System, a blood glucose meter specifically designed for people on multiple daily injections. It may be of help.

☐ Ask to see an insulin pen.

☐ Other: _____.

 Why didn't my math teacher tell me I might need to think like a pancreas?

WEEK
23

The "Work" in Workout

How hard should I exercise?

You should work hard enough to get your body above its resting level. Follow a regular workout schedule at least three times a week to see effects. Avoid consecutive days of hard exercise or a string of consecutive days or weeks with no exercise at all.

Follow your heart . . . rate.

Your heart will tell you if the workout is intense enough to get you positive effects. According to the American Diabetes Association's Standards of Care, adults with diabetes should aim for at least 150 minutes per week of moderate-intensity aerobic physical activity (50–70% of maximum heart rate), spread over at least 3 days per week. You can find the target heart rate for your age by looking at the following chart:

Age	Target heart rate zone
20 years	100–150 beats per minute
25 years	98–146 beats per minute
30 years	95–142 beats per minute
35 years	93–138 beats per minute
40 years	90–135 beats per minute
45 years	88–131 beats per minute
50 years	85–127 beats per minute
55 years	83–123 beats per minute
60 years	80–120 beats per minute
65 years	78–116 beats per minute
70 years	75–113 beats per minute

How do I check my pulse?

Use the index and middle fingers of your dominant hand (your right hand if you're right-handed) to feel the area inside your wrist on your nondominant hand below the base of your thumb (your left hand, if you're right-handed). Count your heartbeats for 10 seconds and multiply that by 6 to get the beats per minute. The next time you see your pharmacist or health-care provider, have them teach you how to check your pulse. If you're feeling particularly modern, you can also buy a heart rate monitor (such as a Polar heart rate monitor at www.polarusa. com or one from Omron at www.omronhealthcare.com).

Or, use the Talk Test

Your ability to talk during exercise will give you a guide as to how hard you are exercising.
- Low intensity: able to sing while exercising
- Moderate intensity: able to speak without gasping while exercising
- Vigorous intensity: winded or too short of breath to talk while exercising

---

PERSONAL GOAL

Date: _____ I will:

☐ Push myself to exercise harder. No one else can do it for me.
☐ Put together a hot playlist or mixtape for my cardio workouts.
☐ Ask my health-care provider to show me how to take my pulse.
☐ Stop exercising if I have chest pain, severe shortness of breath, or leg pain and call my health-care provider immediately.
☐ Inject insulin into an area that I won't use for exercise (e.g., if going running, don't inject into legs).
☐ Increase the intensity, frequency, and duration of my exercise activities.
☐ Other: _____.

 Scooping ice cream is an effective muscular strengthening technique.

Buyer Beware: Glycemic Index

So, what's this glycemic index thing?

You've likely heard of the glycemic index and seen it advertised on products. But what exactly is the glycemic index? Put simply, it measures the body's response to 50 grams of carbohydrate from one kind of food. Sounds helpful, right?

The issue with the glycemic index is that it *does not* measure how rapidly blood glucose levels peak, only how long the glucose will stay in the system. This seems useful, but when was the last time you ate only 50 grams of carbohydrate from one food type? Furthermore, different foods affect different people in different ways. There is no concrete way to say that food A will affect person A the same way as it'll affect person B.

The glycemic index also can be very misleading. For example, potatoes have a higher glycemic index than pizza. Pizza, however, has many more carbohydrates per serving than do potatoes. In the end, you'll get a much higher glucose effect from eating pizza than potatoes, but you wouldn't know that just by looking at the glycemic index. If you're still not confused, consider this: Soft drinks and chocolate candy have a medium glycemic index! Instead, focus on the total carbohydrates you're taking in with each meal.

Food safety

Did you ever get sick from contaminated food? It can send your glucose into orbit. That's why it is important to do the following:

- Clean thoroughly (hands, food, surfaces)
- Keep raw meat, chicken, fish, and eggs separate (in the grocery bag, on cutting boards, on plates, and in the fridge to prevent cross-contamination)

- Cook or microwave food thoroughly
- Chill perishable foods in the refrigerator within 2 hours

PERSONAL GOAL

Date: _____ I will:

☐ Check my glucose before and after my largest meal to understand the carb impact.
☐ Read a new Nutrition Facts label.
☐ Learn more about food safety at www.foodsafety. gov/poisoning/risk/chronicillnesses/index.html.
☐ Other: _____.

 My index finger is pointing at some yummy carbs!

Higher Ground

People frequently underestimate the power that spirituality can bring to their health and wellness, regardless of the form in which that spirituality presents itself. Some examples include faith-based practices (going to church or temple, praying, watching your favorite minister on television, reading scripture, etc.), meditating, being one with nature, journaling, or volunteering. Some religious affiliations offer group diabetes education and support.

Stepping outside of oneself offers positive benefits for diabetes self-management because it can reduce stress levels. We often get caught up in the grind of daily life. Take the time to step away and do something good for your soul.

Have you tried walking a labyrinth? They usually are set up outdoors and have paths that twist and turn to the center and then head back out toward the exit. Walking a labyrinth offers you a way to quiet your mind and awaken your inner wisdom. Many churches, schoolyards, and community centers have them. You can even make your own (see www.labyrinthproject.com).

PERSONAL GOAL

Date: _____ I will:

☐ Develop my own healing rituals.
☐ Find delight in paradox.
☐ Ask people about themselves.
☐ Lighten up on those closest to me.
☐ Spend some quiet time out in the fresh air.
☐ Other: _____.

I'm not lost,
just walking a mental labyrinth.

WEEK 25

Surprise Attacks

What's the connection between diabetes and cardiovascular disease?

People often are shocked to learn that 68% of people with diabetes aged 65 years or older die from heart disease. Insulin resistance is the main issue with type 2 diabetes and is associated with atherosclerosis (the technical name for arteries that are clogged by fatty deposits). When arteries are narrowed, less oxygen can be delivered to the heart and brain. Plaques then can dislodge or create an environment in which blood flow is completely blocked, leading to a heart attack or stroke.

What is a heart attack?

A heart attack occurs when part of the heart muscle dies from lack of oxygen. More than 1 million people in the U.S. have a heart attack (also called a myocardial infarction or MI) every year. It's common to experience angina (temporary chest pain) before having a heart attack (but less likely in people with diabetes, and in women), so it's important to listen to your body's signals. Treatment is aimed at increasing circulation and oxygen back to the heart, thinning blood to prevent clotting, reducing the workload of the heart, and managing blood pressure and cholesterol.

What is a stroke?

A stroke (or cerebral vascular accident or CVA) occurs when the blood flow to an area in the brain stops, either because an artery bursts or is blocked. The number of stroke victims has decreased over the past 45 years thanks to widespread use of medications for high blood pressure and high cholesterol. Women have a higher risk of strokes (1 in 5 women have a stroke) than men (1 in 10).

Depending on the area of the brain that does not get life-sustaining oxygen, the level of destruction can vary from loss of speech and vision to paralysis of a single arm or leg. In the worst cases, strokes result in coma and death. Symptoms include a sudden change in vision, a severe headache, sudden numbness on one side of the body, difficulty understanding what someone just told you, trouble with balance and coordination, and difficulty speaking.

How do I prevent heart attacks and strokes?

Besides following a nutritious diet, being active most days, and maintaining target blood pressure and A1C levels, these steps can further protect your heart and brain:

- Take one baby aspirin tablet (75 or 162 mg) every day if your health-care provider approves it. This is recommended for people with type 1 and 2 diabetes who are at an increased cardiovascular risk (most men older than 50 years of age or women older than 60 years of age who have at least one additional major risk factor: family history of cardiovascular disease, high blood pressure, smoking, high cholesterol, or protein in the urine, called "albuminuria").
- Reduce stress.
- Avoid smoking and secondhand smoke.
- Eat fish three times a week or 1 ounce of walnuts a day to get your dose of protective omega-3s up.
- Improve your cholesterol. Reduce LDL cholesterol by 10% and your risk of heart-related events will go down by 25%. For every 1-milligram increase in HDL cholesterol, the risk for cardiovascular disease drops by 2–3%.
- Have a sleep study done to check for sleep apnea (which is linked to sudden cardiac death and stroke).
- Ask about the need for a cardiac workup (electrocardiogram, stress test).
- Brush and floss your teeth.
- Know your blood pressure and get help in controlling it.

PERSONAL GOAL

Date: _____ I will:

☐ Ask for a referral to a cardiologist who can review my blood pressure.

☐ Seek immediate medical attention for any signs and symptoms of a heart attack or stroke (pain or pressure in the chest, arm, or jaw; dizziness; nausea; shortness of breath; palpitations; fainting; or severe and sudden headache or vision changes).

☐ Ask for help to kick my nicotine addiction and avoid secondhand smoke.

☐ Take my blood pressure medications consistently.

☐ Move my body every day.

☐ Other: _____.

Have a heart and don't tell me
what can go wrong.

WEEK
26

Let Your Cell Phone Help

Better health may be in your hands, thanks to advances in mobile technology via the use of text messages and smartphone applications (or "apps"). If only there was a pancreas app, and you could get on with life. Alas, there is everything but, and new diabetes-related smartphone apps help you track your food, exercise, weight, blood glucose, medications, and insulin dosages, and they will send all of that data to your support network, including your diabetes care providers. Here is a rundown of 10 applications to check out.

	App Name	Device/Platform	Features
1	Glucose Buddy	Works with iPhone, iPod, iPad	Features food, medication and exercise logs, and interactive diabetes education; syncs with your desktop to create charts and graphs to view your health trends.
2	Lose It	Works with iPhone, iPod, iPad	Tracks your calories, carbs, protein, and fat consumption; includes a database of food and recipes; enables users to share progress on Facebook or Twitter!
3	My Fitness Pal	Works with iPhone, iPod, iPad, and BlackBerry, as well as with Android- and Windows-based devices	Available on- and offline; tracks food and exercise; provides fitness ideas and customized plans; enables users to share progress with social networks.
4	dLife Diabetes Companion	Works with iPhone, iPod, iPad	Features easily searchable content from dLife and dLife television; gives you instant access to recipes, reports, expert Q&As, and a tracking system.
5	Nike Training Club	Works with iPhone, iPod, iPad	Almost like having a personal trainer in your phone; provides access to more than 114 customizable workouts.

	App Name	Device/Platform	Features
6	Calorie King	Works with iPhone and iPad	Provides an accurate way to count calories, fat, and carbohydrates in your foods as well as meals in more than 260 fast-food and chain restaurants.
7	Diabetes Health Mobile	Works with any kind of smartphone	Includes articles on the top news and blogs from the Diabetes Health website; sorts information by diabetes type.
8	Diabetes Buddy	Works with iPhone, iPod, iPad	Tracks not just your blood glucose, food, and exercise, but also all the other factors that can influence your diabetes.
9	Go Meals	Works with any kind of smartphone	Provides a massive database for detailed nutritional information in food and dishes from your local grocery stores and restaurants.
10	iBG Star	Works with iPhone, iPod, iPad	Features the first glucose-monitoring system that can connect directly to your Apple device; after attaching the meter to test blood glucose, it tracks carbs, insulin, exercise, and a number of other influencing factors.

PERSONAL GOAL

Date: _____ I will:

☐ Try one of these apps in the previous table.
☐ Sign up for daily diabetes health text messages at www.care4life.com.
☐ Sign up for daily weight-management text messages at www.muschealth.com/WeightMgmtMessaging.
☐ Use this as an excuse to upgrade my cell phone.
☐ Other: _____.

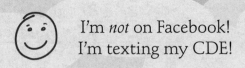

I'm *not* on Facebook!
I'm texting my CDE!

MONTH 6: REVIEW

Date: _____

1. **You started this journey of diabetes self-discovery about 6 months ago. What have you learned about your resilience?**

    _____.

2. Update the status of each of your self-care areas:

- Before-meal blood glucose level averages _____ mg/dL

- 2 hours after-meal blood glucose level averages _____ mg/dL
   (Before-meal target: 70–130 mg/dL; 2 hours after-meal target:
   less than 180 mg/dL)

- Last A1C test result? _____ %
   (Target: less than 7% or estimated glucose average 154 mg/dL)

- Last blood pressure reading _____ mmHg
   (Target: less than 140/80 mmHg)

- Enter my weight: _____

3. When was the last time you:

- Flossed? _____

- Saw the eye doctor? _____

- Talked with your health-care
   provider about your blood pressure?_____

4. How confident do you feel about meal planning and carbohydrate counting for managing your diabetes?

Circle one: Very confident   Somewhat confident   Not confident

(If you do not feel you have a solid grasp on what to eat, please see an RD and a CDE to get the answers.)

5. **Over the past several months, how many days a week on average did you exercise?**

_____ More than 5 days per week

_____ 3–4 days per week

_____ 1–2 days per week

_____ None

_____ I am unable to exercise

6. **Do you feel better equipped to deal with the reality of your diabetes diagnosis?** _____

Why or why not? _____

7. **What was one experience that helped or hurt your self-management efforts most?** _____

_____

8. **Did you take your medication on time?**

Circle one: Nearly always   Sometimes   Almost never

9. **Have you identified humorous situations in everyday moments?**

_____ Yes   _____ No

10. **Go back and identify at least three new goals (from Day 1 through Month 6) that you would like to try:**

1. _____

2. _____

3. _____

MONTH 7

Laughin' Langerhans

By Theresa Garnero

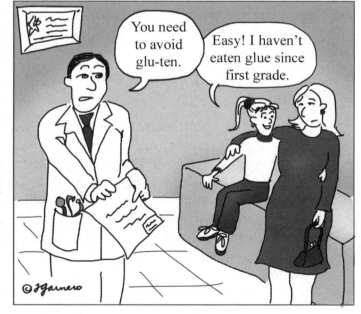

Celebrations

Birthdays, anniversaries, holidays, and other celebrations present a minefield of situations that people with diabetes will have to navigate. With just a little planning, you can prevent turning a joyous occasion into a health-care calamity.

Birthdays

If cake is important, please have *some*. You can exercise earlier in the day or after the dessert, adjust the carbs for your meal, or prepare extra diabetes medication, if needed. Birthdays are special events, so you shouldn't be punished or deprive yourself just because you have diabetes.

Holidays

- **New Year's Eve (December 31).** Always have food with your alcohol. You may need less basal evening insulin should you have champagne on December 31. This can help prevent starting the New Year with hypoglycemia. Carry emergency glucose tablets and a protein bar. You might try a small snack before arriving at a party so you can avoid all-night grazing.
- **Eid al-Adha (the Muslim festival of sacrifice, about 70 days after Ramadan).** Eid al-Adha commemorates Ibrahim's willingness to sacrifice his son for Allah. It concludes with millions of Muslims taking the pilgrimage to Mecca, Saudi Arabia. When sharing two-thirds of your meals with the poor, you will need less insulin and medication due to limited food intake. Consider limiting koftas.
- **Chinese New Year (varies, end of January to mid-February).** Traditions require people to practice various customs

that promote prosperity (sharing tangerines or oranges to symbolize abundant happiness) and ward off bad spirits (lighting firecrackers and wearing red). This week-long celebration is filled with all kinds of carbs. Be careful when it comes to the togetherness candy tray. Pace yourself and share money-filled red envelopes instead.

- **Easter (varies, late March to late April).** If you're fasting for church service, you may need to reduce or hold off on your morning diabetes medications (check with your health-care provider first); pass on the chocolate bunny ears.
- **Ramadan (Islamic month of fasting, dates change, about 13 days earlier each consecutive year).** People with diabetes are not required or advised to fast. If you wish to fast, get an individualized plan together with your care provider to accommodate the predawn to sunset fast to prevent hypoglycemia, hyperglycemia, and dehydration.
- **Thanksgiving (fourth Thursday of November).** Bring a healthy choice to share, have a little of each dish instead of a lot, build exercise into the day, and ask about the best medicine approach to take.
- **Bodhi Day (Buddha's Enlightenment, December 8).** Choose a small portion of rice and milk, count your carbs, and act accordingly. Consider adding a protein. If meditating for hours, you may need less medicine and a way to prevent dehydration.
- **Virgin of Guadalupe feast day (honors the patron saint of Mexico, December 12).** Adjust medicines to handle the several hours of morning fasting followed with high-carb foods (champurrado, tamales, and sweet bread). You may need less evening insulin or to hold off on your morning medications until you have food and additional fast-acting insulin to cover the extra carbs. Bring a sugar source, so you will be prepared if you start to feel dizzy or low.
- **Hanukkah (Jewish Festival of Lights, various dates, normally 8 days in December).** Enjoy the stuffed beef brisket or fowl. Try baking potato latkes instead of frying them. Try challah bread made from whole wheat instead of egg-enriched yeast, and limit the honey-sweetened desserts. Plan for extra walking or extra medications to combat the extra carbs.
- **Christmas (December 25).** Bring a carbohydrate source with

you to church services, as lows can occur in the middle of a service. You also can accept all neighborly gifts of baked goods to share with your friends and family. Have a snack if the main feast is delayed. You may need more bolus insulin to account for the big meal. Ask for donations to be made to the American Diabetes Association for diabetes research rather than giving you a gift.

- **Boxing Day/St. Stephen's Day (December 26, in most cases).** Go easy on buffet lines. Fish around for the dime in the plum pudding and limit the cream. All of the other tips about alcohol and exercise apply here, too!
- **Kwanzaa (African American/Pan-African celebration, December 26 to January 1).** Have the karamu (yams, sesame seeds, collard greens, and hot peppers) early in the evening if you also plan to celebrate New Year's Eve. Factor the candied yams into your bolus insulin dose. Watch your alcohol intake in the passing of a communal unity cup.

PERSONAL GOAL

Date: _____ I will:

☐ Check with my health-care provider about adjusting my medications for periods of fasting.
☐ Carry glucose tablets and a protein bar.
☐ Exercise before a feast.
☐ Sample a little of everything instead of the second helpings.
☐ Politely accept baked gifts and pass them on.
☐ Periodically check my blood glucose during celebrations.
☐ Other: _____.

 When can I send my diabetes on an all-expenses-paid vacation?

How do I know whether my meter is accurate?

It's common to second guess your meter's accuracy when a glucose result doesn't make sense. Even though today's glucose meters are leaps and bounds better than the old methods (urine test strips), a variety of factors can affect the accuracy of a glucose meter. Here is a short list of possible explanations for an unexpected reading.

The International Organization for Standardization (ISO) recommends minimum acceptable meter accuracy (within ±15% above or below the lab value; that is, they have done simultaneous testing to compare glucose results from meters versus venipuncture blood draws). The ISO figures, based on device testing, do not guarantee results or protect against common user errors.

With this standard, a glucose meter reading of 300 mg/dL can actu-

Measure My Meter

- Test strip: type (avoid third-party, generic ones; see the note on ISO standards, above), age (freshness, old or expired), storage (kept in an airtight container, not exposing strip to light or air)
- Dirty hands (food or glucose tablet residual on fingertips hence the important to wash hands before checking)
- Size of blood sample (don't oversqueeze your finger to get enough blood for a sample)
- Environmental conditions: temperature, climate, and altitude
- Percentage of red blood cells in the blood, or hematocrit level (anemia, sickle cell anemia, and kidney failure can affect hematocrit levels)
- Debris or buildup of dried blood where the strip enters the meter
- Low batteries
- Meter calibration (on older models)
- Interfering substances in one's blood from medications (now rare, but something as simple as Tylenol used to be an issue; new systems correct for this problem. Check the fine print on your meter instruction booklet or call the toll-free number to ask about any interfering medications)
- Severe dehydration can result in false high readings
- Alternative site testing (sites other than the fingertips can have differing glucose levels)

ally be a plasma value between 255 and 345 mg/dL. If you take insulin to correct the "300 mg/dL" reading, the final glucose will vary as your "true" starting value could have been as low as 255 or as high as 345 mg/dL. Some meters help to reduce this variable by exceeding the ISO standard by being within 10% above or below lab values. This is just another variable to appreciate. The important point is to be consistent with your technique to maximize the consistency within your results and the actions you take. It is still light years ahead of the accuracy of urine glucose testing.

Why is this so complicated?

Glucose meters measure electrical currents! What? As described by blogger Amy Tenderich, glucose interacts with an enzyme on the strip, releasing electrons. Another agent on the strip, called the "mediator," turns these electrons into an electrical current. The greater the glucose concentration, the greater the current. That current then speeds through the strip. Finally, an algorithm (formula) in the meter converts the current into a concentration of glucose. And voilà! You get a number.

When you test your glucose twice on the same meter a minute apart, you will get a different number. Why? The first drop of blood you squeeze out of your finger is not the same as the very next drop of blood, and as such, the electrical current (as described previously) will be different. It also may contain more interstitial fluid (the solution that surrounds your cells), which can give a lower reading. And then there is the variability in how the meter interprets the data.

Running a control solution test

Some manufacturers include a glucose control solution (water with a controlled amount of sugar) with their meters. You can run this test if you question your meter's accuracy or if something happened to your meter (like dropping it down a flight of stairs). How? Insert a strip in the meter and place a drop of the glucose control solution onto the test strip. Check to see whether the result is within range for the control solution (usually written on the bottle, or on the vial of strips). If it matches the correct range, then your meter is working fine. If not, call the meter company.

Involve your health-care provider

Bring your meter and readings to your health-care provider. It helps to identify patterns to come up with solutions. If you do not have a meter, ask for help in selecting the best one. If you have one and don't like it, ask about other options.

PERSONAL GOAL

Date: _____ I will:

☐ Make sure my hands are clean before I check my glucose level.
☐ Call the toll-free number on the back of the meter to ask any questions and for troubleshooting help.
☐ Check the expiration date on the test strips.
☐ Keep the meter and strips away from extreme temperatures.
☐ Other: _____.

This call may be monitored for quality glucose control.

WEEK
28

 Muscle Fitness

Resistance or strength training builds muscle mass. Muscles burn more calories than fat, even when you're not exercising. Your muscle fitness helps you maintain or lose weight, manage blood glucose levels, improve balance and posture, and minimize the risk for injury. You can accomplish all of this through resistance exercises and weight training.

What is resistance training?

Resistance training uses exercises that fatigue the muscles by using your body as a weight (e.g., leg squats and push-ups), by using minimal equipment (e.g., hand weights, jump ropes, elastic bands, balance balls), or by using the machine equipment found in most gyms.

Safety is the first step

Before you grab those dumbbells, consider the following safety tips:
- Warm up for 5 minutes by walking on the treadmill, jumping rope, or doing gentle jumping jacks.
- Stretch your muscles when they are warmed up, not cold.
- If you have high blood pressure and are just starting your activity program, exercise at only 50% of your maximum heart rate and gradually build up to 75%.
- Give your muscles 1 or 2 days off between resistance or strength training exercises (do a different type of activity on alternate days).
- When lifting weights, exhale when lifting or pushing and inhale when lowering or relaxing the muscles.
- Ask your health-care provider for a referral to an exercise professional with experience in working with people with diabetes. An exercise physiologist or specialized provider can help develop an individualized exercise program for you.

The basics of resistance training

These basics only skim the surface of resistance training, but they should be sufficient to get you started. Begin with an exercise that lets you move in a smooth manner repeating that same movement (known as "repetitions" or "reps"). Do two sets of 10 repetitions (known as a "set") with a short rest (about 1 minute) between sets.

Over time, increase the sets to five. When working with weights or exercise equipment that allows you to adjust the tension (such as treadmills, stationary bikes, and stair steppers), begin with the easiest setting or weight. Do the exercise slowly and stay in control of your muscles.

Your mission is to challenge and fatigue your muscles, not pull a muscle or cause a herniated disc. As you become familiar with resistance training, and with your health-care provider's guidance, you can modify your approach to meet your personal goals:

- **To increase your muscle strength,** gradually increase the weight and decrease the repetitions (to eight).
- **To increase muscle endurance and toning,** use lighter weights and increase repetitions (up to 20).

Examples of workout components include the following:

- Leg squats and side leg raises (two sets of 10 repetitions)
- Wall sit (two sets of 30 seconds)
- Standing push-ups: place hands on a sturdy wall, a little wider than shoulder-width apart; keeping your torso and neck straight, lower yourself toward the wall going as low as possible without it touching your chest; return to starting position (two sets of 10)
- Leg lunges with 2- to 5-pound weights (two sets of 10 repetitions, each side)
- Bicep curls with no weights or 1- to 5-pound weights or resistance bands (two sets of 10 repetitions)
- Shoulder press: hold a bottle of water in each hand at about ear level; press weights up and over your head; bring back down to just above the shoulder (two sets of 10 repetitions)
- Torso twists (*gentle* rotations; two sets of 15 repetitions)
- Leg press at the gym (two sets of 8 repetitions)
- Bicep curls at the gym (two sets of 8 repetitions)
- Triceps extensions at the gym (two sets of 8 repetitions)

PERSONAL GOAL

Date: _____ I will:

☐ Ask my health-care provider to review what exercises are safe for me.

☐ Try one of the above strengthening exercises every other day this week.

☐ Challenge my muscles.

☐ Other: _____.

 My muscles are giving me a fit.

Those Pesky Pesticides

If I'm eating fruits and vegetables, isn't that good enough?

Pat yourself on the back if you've managed to incorporate fresh fruits and vegetables as a regular part of your diet. Be aware, however, that you may be consuming pesticides along with these foods. According to the Environmental Working Group, pesticides can cause health problems, and thus it is possible to lower your dietary pesticide load by rinsing all of your produce, eating a varied diet, and buying organic *when possible*. In one study, the researchers found a strong dose–response relation between serum concentrations of persistent organic pollutants and diabetes. You don't have to buy organic; there are plenty of conventionally grown options as you consider this controversial topic.

Best to buy organic—These items had the highest pesticide load:	Okay to buy conventionally grown—These foods had the lowest pesticide load:
Apples	Onions
Celery	Sweet corn
Sweet bell peppers	Pineapples
Peaches	Avocado
Strawberries	Cabbage
Spinach	Sweet peas
Nectarines (imported)	Asparagus
Grapes	Mangoes
Spinach	Eggplant
Lettuce	Kiwi
Cucumbers	Cantaloupe (domestic)
Blueberries (domestic)	Sweet potatoes
Potatoes	Grapefruit
Green beans	Watermelon
Kale/collard greens	Mushrooms

PERSONAL GOAL

Date: _____ I will:

☐ Copy this list to keep handy.
☐ Wash all produce.
☐ Enjoy an eggplant dish.
☐ Go to a local farmer's market (search at www. organicconsumers.org).
Other: _____.

WEEK
30

Weight-Loss Options When Lifestyle Changes Aren't Enough

Bariatric surgery

Mainstream diabetes organizations support the use of bariatric surgery—a procedure that alters the stomach—for people with a BMI between 30 and 35 or more (which is reported as kg/m²), and whose type 2 diabetes can't be controlled adequately, particularly when other cardiovascular risk factors are present.

There are two main procedure types: restrictive (reducing the size of the stomach, which makes a person feel full after a few bites) and malabsorptive (rearranging the plumbing of the stomach in such a way that leads to reduced appetite).

This may seem extreme, but it has helped many people to lose significant weight, lower cardiovascular risk, and, for some, achieve remission of type 2 diabetes. Six years after gastric bypass surgery, diabetes remission for extremely overweight (called morbidly obese) individuals was 75%. People with more than 5 years of type 2 diabetes before bariatric surgery were 3.8 times more likely to have diabetes recur. Gastric surgery remains impractical for millions of eligible adults, and it is not without complications (like infection or hypoglycemia).

In 2013, the FDA approved a new weight-loss drug called Belviq (lorcaserin HCL) for use as an adjunct to a reduced-caloric diet and increased physical activity for chronic weight management for adults with an initial BMI of 30 kg/m² or greater (obese), or a BMI of 27 kg/m² or greater (overweight) in the presence of at least one weight-related associated condition (type 2 diabetes, high blood pressure or high cholesterol).

If you think this procedure or medication could be of benefit, discuss it at your next medical appointment.

PERSONAL GOAL

Date: _____ I will:

☐ I will do the following for my waistline:

_____

_____

_____

_____.

MONTH 8

Laughin' Langerhans   By Theresa Garnero

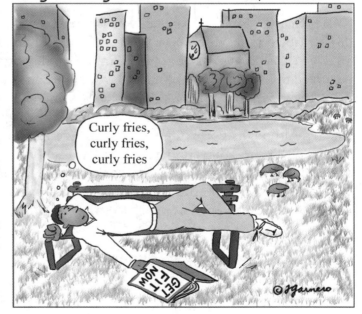

WEEK
31

Going Gluten-Free

What is gluten?

Gluten is a protein found in wheat, barley, and rye—common ingredients in food and beverages. Have you noticed a new section in your grocery store devoted to gluten-free foods? It has been growing as research and awareness about gluten intolerance are on the rise.

Should I go gluten-free?

The main reason to go gluten-free is if you have an autoimmune disease called celiac disease, which results in an inability to digest gluten because of damage to the villi in the small intestine and can be linked to countless symptoms. Classic symptoms include bloating, diarrhea, abdominal pain, and weight loss, while others may be unrelated to your gastrointestinal system, making the diagnosis extra challenging. Although approximately 1% of the general population and people with type 2 diabetes have celiac disease, 10% of people with type 1 diabetes have it. Celiac disease can be diagnosed through blood tests, although the gold standard for diagnosis is a biopsy of your small intestine done in an endoscopy.

100%? Can't I be just 99% gluten-free?

That depends. If you have celiac disease, it is critical to be 100% gluten-free. Just 1/100th of a piece of toast is enough gluten to set off your autoimmune response. This means that you need to be careful with sharing a toaster or cooking materials with someone who is eating gluten, to avoid any cross-contamination. You'll also need to look out for hidden gluten in products, such as makeup, mouthwash, medications, vitamins, and even rubber bands.

Life without gluten

Ridding your life of gluten may seem like a daunting task. But if gluten is causing unpleasant symptoms or damaging your intestines as in the case of celiac disease, the payoff is worth it. Still, some people who can't eat gluten feel frustrated, isolated, upset, or overwhelmed at various times. You already are wrapping your mind around the diabetes diagnosis and going gluten-free can feel like the last straw. Remember to reach out to your support network and your health-care team. You can see a dietitian who is knowledgeable about both diabetes and gluten-free diets. There are lots of interesting and varied meals you can make that are both diabetes-friendly and gluten-free.

PERSONAL GOAL

Date: _____ I will:

☐ Ask my health-care provider for the celiac disease blood test at my next appointment.

☐ Eat a gluten-free food that I haven't tried before.

☐ Visit the National Foundation for Celiac Awareness at www. celiaccentral.org.

☐ Go to www.csaceliacs.org to search for a local celiac disease support group.

☐ Other: _____.

 How about an autoimmune disease that puts me on a celery-free diet?

WEEK
32

Get with the Program: At Home

Have you thought about getting your dose of exercise in the comfort and convenience of your own home? It can be relatively easy to convert a small area in your home into a workout space.

There are benefits to having a home exercise program. It's easier on your wallet, and fewer variables interfere with making it happen (weather, body image concerns, time to commute to the gym, etc.).

Sounds great, but how do I do it?

Here are two great ways to bring exercise into your own home.

1. **Videos.** Choose an exercise or activity you enjoy and look for a video to guide you.
   - Satellite television offers many exercise programs.
   - Collage Video is a company that offers every kind of exercise video under the sun, all of which are reviewed by an instructor certified by the American Council on Exercise. Previews and customer reviews of videos are available on their website (www.collagevideo.com).

2. **Invest in a home gym.** You can get fit if you know the right equipment to buy. If you choose this option, be sure to do a lot of research to be sure that you're buying safe, reliable machinery.

PERSONAL GOAL

Date: _____ I will:

☐ Make a plan to exercise at home.
☐ Lay out my exercise clothes the night before my morning workout.
☐ Contact a local gym or exercise equipment store to try out equipment before I buy it.
☐ Find out warranty and return information.
☐ Other: _____.

 A gym in my house? Why, so I can feel guilty every time I come home?

The Nerve of Neuropathy

Nerves communicate information about pain, temperature, and touch directly to your brain. If you burn your hand on the stove, your nervous system sends that message at lightning speed to the brain and you pull your hand away without thinking about it. Nerves also help with digestion, bladder function, sexual function, sweating, detection of low glucose levels, and the warning signs of a heart attack.

What is diabetic neuropathy?

Diabetic neuropathy is nerve damage that occurs as a result of uncontrolled blood glucose levels. Neuropathy occurs in nearly half of all people with diabetes and can result in pain or loss of sensation.

How do I know if I really have diabetic neuropathy?

Your health-care provider will look at your complete medical picture with a careful history and physical examination. You should be screened annually for diabetic peripheral neuropathy with tests performed at the office visit. These include the pinprick sensation test (the painless little metal wheel with spokes), the vibration sensation test (using

What Are the Symptoms of Neuropathy?

- Tingling, burning, or stabbing pains in the feet or hands that are typically worse at night and sensitive to the touch.
- Very cold or very hot feet or hands.
- Feeling like you are wearing socks or gloves when you aren't.
- Numb or extremely dry feet.
- Weak and unsteady leg muscles.
- Difficulty balancing when walking.
- Frequent indigestion or nausea.
- Vomiting undigested food (a sign of gastroparesis).
- Feeling bloated or full after very little food.
- Frequent diarrhea or constipation.
- Bladder issues (frequent leakage, infections, urge to go with very little results).
- Sexual problems (trouble getting aroused or reaching orgasm).
- Fast heartbeat while at rest.
- Dizziness when standing.
- No warning signs of low blood glucose.
- Sweating when eating certain foods.

a tuning fork), a monofilament pressure test (piece of plastic used to touch your toes to see if you can feel it), and checking ankle reflexes. If you are having problems, your health-care provider may refer you to a neurologist (a doctor who specializes in nerves).

What are the treatments for diabetic neuropathy?

Following are some treatment options for diabetic neuropathy:

- **Medication.** Many medications help address and minimize the symptoms of neuropathy. Talk with your health-care provider about the best one for you because most treatment methods do include a risk of side effects. Options include anti-depressants (used in lower doses than those for people with depression), anticonvulsants (reduces the pain of neuropathy), topical creams (sometimes used to treat neuropathy in specific locations), narcotic analgesics (serious painkillers for really bad pain), and anesthetics.
- **Transcutaneous electrical nerve stimulation (TENS).** TENS delivers tiny electrical impulses along specific nerve pathways through small pads placed on your skin. This may help prevent pain signals from reaching the brain. It's safe and virtually painless. Its effectiveness varies based on the type and severity of the neuropathy.
- **Biofeedback.** Biofeedback therapy uses a special machine that teaches you how to control your responses to pain.
- **Monochromatic infrared therapy (Anodyne therapy).** This treatment method uses beams of infrared light to treat neuropathy. The infrared light goes through the skin over the affected area, causes the release of nitric oxide from red blood cells, helps circulation, and improves nerve conduction. Learn more at www.anodynetherapy.com.
- **Surgery.** Surgical nerve decompression is a procedure that frees the nerve pathways that typically get entrapped in specific areas. Plastic surgeons perform this as an outpatient procedure, and it cures the neuropathy most of the time.

If you have diabetes,
sometimes it gets on your nerves.

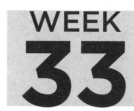
 Glucose and Blood Pressure Review

Let's look at the state of your blood glucose and blood pressure levels.

Blood glucose levels

Checking your blood glucose levels has a huge effect on your A1C values, as long as you know what to do with the results.

1. **How often do you check?**
   ☐ Daily, at varied times (before and 2 hours after meals)
   ☐ Daily, at one time of the day (e.g., morning only)
   ☐ A few times a week
   ☐ Weekly
   ☐ Rarely
   ☐ My meter isn't working
   ☐ I'm not testing (for whatever reason)
   ☐ Other: _____

2. **What is your premeal average (more than half of the time)?**
   ☐ Less than 70 mg/dL (see question 3)
   ☐ 71–130 mg/dL (this is the goal)
   ☐ 131–160 mg/dL
   ☐ 161–200 mg/dL
   ☐ 201 mg/dL and above

3. **How many lows (less than 70 mg/dL) have you had this week?** _____.
   Call your health-care provider if you have more than two readings of less than 70 mg/dL within 1 week.

4. **Most of the time, what is your 2-hour after-meal range?**
   ☐ Less than 180 mg/dL (this is the goal)
   ☐ 181– 240 mg/dL
   ☐ 241 mg/dL and above

5. **If your glucose is not in the target range most of the time or if you are experiencing readings of less than 70 mg/dL more than twice a week, does your health-care provider know?**
   ☐ Yes ☐ No

6. **If you have involved your health-care provider, has your treatment changed?**
   ☐ Yes ☐ No

7. **If your blood glucose patterns are still outside the target range despite multiple medication adjustments, has your health-care provider referred you to a specialist (such as an endocrinologist or a diabetologist)?**
   ☐ Yes ☐ No

8. **What was your last A1C result?**
   _____ % (target is less than 7%)   Date taken: _____

Blood pressure levels

Time to put the pressure on about bringing your blood pressure down!

9. **How often do you check your blood pressure?**
   ☐ Daily, at various times
   ☐ Daily, in the morning
   ☐ A few times a week
   ☐ Rarely
   ☐ Only at my health-care provider's office
   ☐ I don't have blood pressure monitoring equipment
   ☐ Other: _____

10. What is your average blood pressure reading?

Systolic (top number)	Diastolic (bottom number)
Less than 130 mmHg (target)	Less than 80 mmHg (target)
131–140 mmHg	81–90 mmHg
141–150 mmHg	91–100 mmHg
151–160 mmHg	101–110 mmHg
161–170 mmHg	111–120 mmHg
171–180 mmHg	121–130 mmHg
181 mmHg and above	131 mmHg and above
Other: _____	Other: _____

11. If you have involved your health-care provider, has your blood pressure treatment changed?

☐ Yes ☐ No

12. If your blood pressure patterns are still above target despite multiple medication adjustments, has your health-care provider referred you to a specialist (such as a cardiologist)?

☐ Yes ☐ No

PERSONAL GOAL

Date: _____ I will:

☐ Check my blood glucose at times when I normally don't test.
☐ Send my blood glucose data to my health-care provider (by fax, e-mail, or phone).
☐ Ask my health-care provider for a new treatment plan for problematic blood glucose or blood pressure patterns.
☐ Other: _____.

 My blood pressure and blood glucose meters chipped in for me to have a massage.

Test the Waters

Test the glucose and jump in—the water's warm!

Showers, baths, and hot tubs

If you have lost any nerve sensation and cannot feel the difference between hot and cold, test the water temperature on an area that can (like your elbow or wrist). People have burned themselves by getting into a scalding bath or shower (when the water heater thermostat was set way too high).

Pools

Check your blood glucose before taking the plunge, swim with others, and have snacks nearby. Follow these precautions and you should be fine.

Oceans, creeks, and rivers

In addition to the obvious risks that come with the power of water, beware of potentially harmful concentrations of microorganisms in crowded waters. These parasites and spores are highest when the beaches and rivers are busiest, and they can cause vomiting and diarrhea. If you are not feeling your best, pass on getting into a crowded waterway.

Cruises

Feel like a relaxing vacation cruise? Tell your travel agent you have diabetes when you book your trip. Most cruises offer a wide variety of food choices.

PERSONAL GOAL

Date: _____ I will:

☐ Check my water heater thermostat and turn it down to a safe level.
☐ Check the water and my blood glucose before I hot tub or go for a swim.
☐ Have juice next to my bath or hot tub in case I feel low.
☐ Other: _____.

Surfboards now come in grape glucose tablet flavor, just in case surf's up and my glucose is down.

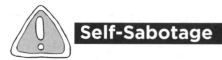

Cocaine and amphetamines

Cocaine and amphetamines were popular in the 1980s, and they remain deadly in the new millennium. Cocaine and amphetamines can make your blood glucose levels look like a rocket shooting skyward and can be deadly. They put a tremendous amount of stress on your heart and liver. If you do have a habit with these drugs, find support to stop immediately.

Marijuana

Marijuana use can increase insulin resistance, impair judgment, and give you a case of the munchies, which brings unwanted calories into your diet. Aside from the smoking issue (or even if you use a vaporizer), marijuana use can increase your need for insulin, worsen your blood glucose control due to overeating, and affect your ability to successfully manage blood glucose highs and lows. Research, however, into a compound found in medicinal cannabis called cannabidiol (CBD) has shown some unexpected effects in limited testing (i.e., it may prevent type 1 diabetes in mice). CBD does not make people feel "stoned," but nonetheless, it remains highly controversial.

Prescription Pain Medicines

In 2010, approximately 16 million Americans reported using a prescription drug for nonmedical reasons in the past year. Some of the intoxication effects are the same symptoms of high and low blood glucose, such as drowsiness, weakness, dry mouth, sweating, and dizziness. Because many of these drugs and diabetes medications are processed in the liver, and people with type 2 diabetes are at a higher risk for nonalcoholic fatty liver disease (something your provider will screen for with yearly labs), don't take a chance. If you take prescription pain medicine when you are not in pain, get help and support in learning how to safely withdraw.

Tobacco

Smoking was discussed at length earlier, but it is worth noting again the dangers it poses to people with diabetes. If you smoke, get help and support in quitting.

PERSONAL GOAL

Date: _____ I will:

☐ Admit I am struggling with a substance abuse problem.
☐ Turn down invitations to try a new drug.
☐ Quit smoking (cigarettes, cigars, or joints); quit chewing tobacco.
☐ Say I'm sorry to someone I hurt with my drug-related behavior.
☐ Take a step toward cleaning my body of a toxic addiction.
☐ Check out Alcoholics Anonymous (AA) at www.alcoholicsanonymous.org or look for a local AA program.
☐ Check out Narcotics Anonymous at www.na.org.
☐ Seek counseling about my prescription drug use.
☐ Other: _____.

Do you abuse prune juice?

MONTH 9

Laughin' Langerhans

By Theresa Garnero

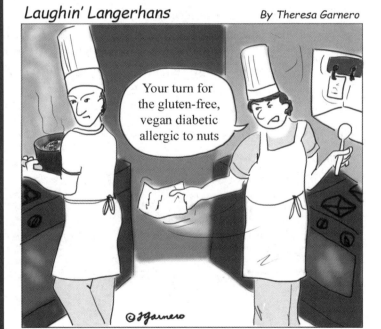

Amylinomimetics: Symlin (Pramlintide Acetate)

Who takes this drug?

Symlin is prescribed for people with type 1 or type 2 diabetes who require insulin.

What is Symlin?

The pancreas simultaneously releases the hormones insulin (from the beta-cells) and amylin (from the alpha-cells). Insulin and amylin work together to help control glucose, especially after meals. The synthetic version of amylin is Symlin. Like insulin, Symlin must be injected. *Never mix the two in the same syringe.*

How does Symlin work?

Symlin helps slow gastric emptying, which helps control the rate at which glucose is absorbed into the bloodstream. This in turn reduces appetite and may result in weight loss. It also reduces the glucose released from the liver. Symlin often reduces the amount of insulin that is required by people who inject it. One disadvantage is the increase in number of injections required. The flip side, however, is that it can help reduce unpredictable swings in blood glucose levels and improve overall diabetes control.

Possible side effects

Because Symlin lowers blood glucose levels, insulin dosages will need to be reduced or else there is an increased risk of hypoglycemia. Because Symlin slows the rate of digestion, the effectiveness of other medications taken by mouth may be affected.

Warning

Symlin is not recommended for women who are pregnant or breast-feeding.

PERSONAL GOAL

Date: _____ I will:

☐ Ask my health-care provider about detailed instructions on how to slowly increase or decrease my Symlin dose.

☐ Agree to skip my Symlin injection if I have hypoglycemia before a meal, do not plan to eat, have less than 250 calories or less than 30 grams of carbohydrate at a meal, am sick and can't eat my usual meal, or am going to have surgery or a medical test where I cannot eat beforehand.

☐ Other: _____.

Amy-Lynn . . . a hormone named after my teenage daughter.

The Skinny on Skin Care

Skin is your personal homeland security system—it protects the body from dangerous environmental elements (bacteria, chemicals, the sun's ultraviolet rays), including heat and cold. It's the largest organ in the body, weighing about 25 pounds, and is one of our most versatile organs, regulating body temperature, preventing loss of essential body fluids, and getting rid of toxic substances with sweat.

How does diabetes affect my skin?

In the short term, high glucose levels pull water from the skin cells and may cause the skin to be dry or feel itchy or sore. This may lead to cracked skin and worse. A simple scratch or break in the skin can cause an infection. In the long term, high glucose levels can cause the tiny blood vessels near the skin to narrow or even clog, further increasing the risk of infection.

People with diabetes have higher rates of psoriasis, a condition that affects the skin and joints. Psoriasis causes red, raised areas of dry skin, often seen on the elbows and knees, but it can affect any area of skin. Psoriasis can cause a type of arthritis and create an increased risk for heart attacks in people with diabetes. Protect yourself by getting treatment for high blood pressure and high cholesterol and by quitting smoking or reducing your exposure to secondhand smoke.

PERSONAL GOAL

Date: _____ I will:

☐ Protect myself from getting minor scratches in my skin (watch out for pets, garden shrubs, long fingernails, splinters) and wear shoes.

☐ After bathing, I'll dry myself well (especially under the breasts, the groin area, and between the toes).

☐ Check my skin after each bath or shower to look for any red or sore spots.

☐ Use fragrance-free lotion to keep my skin moist (but not between my toes).

☐ Use SPF-15 sunscreen daily.

☐ Call my skin doctor (dermatologist) for help with any skin issues I'm having.

☐ Other: _____.

 With sunscreen, shades, and a helmet, I can finally leave the house.

Being Active with Physical Limitations

The talk of exercise and its benefits can be a downer if you have physical limitations that prevent you from getting regular activity. Whether you have pain, arthritis, or weakness from the aftermath of a stroke, or are unsteady on your feet, chair exercises may be the ticket to increased stamina, muscle strength, and improved blood glucose control.

With a little guidance, you can move your body in a comfortable and effective way to improve flexibility and coordination. You also can do chair exercises while watching television. Check out the award-winning Armchair Fitness videos that complement each other for a complete fitness program.

PERSONAL GOAL

Date: _____ I will:

☐ Visit Armchair Fitness Videos (www.armchairfitness.com) or call 1-800-453-6280.

☐ Check out the "Sit and Be Fit" videos from Collage Video by visiting www.collagevideo.com.

☐ Ask my health-care provider or physical therapist about exercise programs with dynamic chair exercises.

☐ Sign up for a water exercise program (takes the stress off joints).

☐ Other: _____.

Great—you've ruined how I look at my recliner.

WEEK
37

 Dental Health Checkup

If you've been following along, you'll know that 6 months have passed, and it's time for a dental health checkup.

Answer these questions and then pick a new goal for dental health:

1. How many times did you floss this past week? _____
2. When was the last time you flossed? _____
3. When was the last time you replaced your toothbrush? _____

PERSONAL GOAL

Date: _____ I will:

☐ Make an appointment to see my dental hygienist.

☐ Report any tooth or gum problems to my dentist.

☐ Buy products with the American Dental Association's Seal of Acceptance (advertising claims are scientifically supported).

☐ Ask my pharmacist if any of my medications could cause dry mouth.

☐ Rinse my mouth with water immediately after meals.

☐ Ask my dentist about toothpaste specially formulated for dry mouth (e.g., Biotene).

☐ Other: _____.

Want to give your fingers a rest from being pricked for all of that blood glucose monitoring? Alternate site testing may be the ticket.

Your fingertips have more nerve endings than the forearm. Many people feel that alternate site testing hurts less than the traditional side-of-the-finger route, and this method is ideal for some professions, such as musicians, computer techs, health-care workers, and environmental engineers.

The amount of blood required to perform an alternate site test is minimal. Because of decreased circulation in the arm, however, you may need to rub your arm before using the lancet device to get an adequate blood sample and obtain accurate results.

How do I know if I should use alternate site testing?

Try it once to see if you like it. Following are the factors to consider:

- **Your body hair.** Too much makes it tough to get a drop of blood.
- **Access to alternate sites.** Do you wear long sleeves that could make it difficult to get to your arm?
- **You bruise or bleed easily.** A pinprick may turn into a bloody mess that is difficult to cover with a bandage.

Can I use alternate site testing all the time?

No, you cannot use alternate site testing during periods of rapid fluctuations in blood glucose. The arm responds to glucose levels more slowly than the fingertip. You might feel low and test your arm, but the low reading hasn't made it to your arm yet. Do not use alternate site testing if you:

- Have a history of hypoglycemia unawareness (you don't know when you are low).
- Think your blood glucose is low.
- Check after exercise (you won't get an accurate reading from an alternate site).

When in doubt, always test on the fingertip.

PERSONAL GOAL

Date: _____ I will:

☐ Find out whether my meter has an alternate site testing option and whether I have the right equipment (sometimes a different lancet device or attachment is required).
☐ Rub the alternate site to increase circulation before checking my blood glucose levels.
☐ Avoid alternate site testing if I feel low, if I just finished exercising, or if I don't feel well.
☐ Other: _____.

Use someone else for your alternate site test.

WEEK
38

 Achoo! The Flu and You

What's the fuss over the flu?

When the flu enters the picture and you have diabetes, your chances of getting seriously ill are much greater than those of the general population. If you get the flu, you can face complications, potential hospitalization, and, much worse, death. An ounce of prevention can save your life. Getting the flu shot, frequently washing your hands, and avoiding touching your face during flu season are the best ways to reduce your chances of catching the flu.

When should I get vaccinated?

As long as your health-care professional has cleared you for a flu shot, you probably should get it during the fall. If you miss that window, find out whether it's okay to get one later because the flu season can last into spring. Encourage family members to get vaccinated, too.

Where can I get a vaccination?

You can get one from your health-care provider and sometimes at local health fairs or pharmacies.

Helpful Prevention Reminders

- Avoid exposure to the flu by staying away from people with it.
- Wash hands regularly.
- Build resistance and ability to fend off illness by eating healthfully, staying fit, and getting plenty of rest.
- Stay home when sick.
- If you don't see your health-care providers wash their hands, ask if they did.
- Cover your mouth and nose when sneezing or coughing.

PERSONAL GOAL

Date: _____ I will:

☐ Wash my hands frequently.
☐ Get the flu vaccination if it's fall or mark my calendar to remind myself and my family to have one.
☐ Get the pneumonia shot at my next appointment if I've never had one and I'm less than 65 years old, and remember to get another one after age 65 years.
☐ Clean my work area (phone and keyboard) with antiseptic wipes.
☐ If I get the flu, stay hydrated, check my blood glucose every few hours, and call my health-care provider as needed.
☐ Other: _____.

Where's the vaccine to prevent getting cupcake cravings?

WEEK
39

 Me Time

When was the last time you did something nice for yourself? Was it this week? This month? Do you do it on a regular basis? Do you find yourself in a give–give–give mode from dawn until dusk? We tend to put work, family, and other obligations first. Try to give yourself just 15 minutes. You're worth it.

PERSONAL GOAL

Date: _____ I will:

☐ Meditate.

☐ Take a 20-minute nap.

☐ Make an appointment to get a massage (it releases neurochemicals that prompt relaxation, which in turn will can lower blood pressure and blood glucose; plus, it feels really good).

☐ Buy a small acupressure roller or foot massaging tool to help me relax and boost my energy.

☐ Listen to my favorite relaxing music for at least 5 minutes.

☐ Add a few drops of essential lavender oil to my baths for the calming effects of aromatherapy (try mint, lemon, or pine scents for a refreshing effect).

☐ Schedule something I enjoy.

☐ Other: _____.

 If I can't say nice things to myself,
I won't say anything at all!

MONTH 9: REVIEW

Date: _____

You were hit with this diagnosis about 9 months ago. How are you feeling? What have you changed? What have you liked as a result of the change? Who can you reach out to for extra support? How have you been able to help others in your circle?

_____

_____

_____

_____

_____

_____

_____

_____

_____

_____

_____

_____

_____

_____

_____

_____

_____

MONTH 10

Laughin' Langerhans

By Theresa Garnero

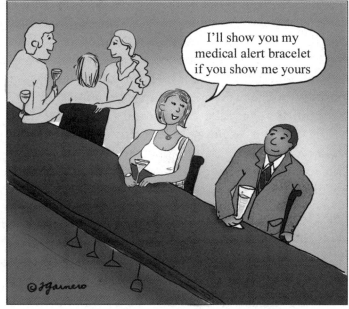

WEEK 40

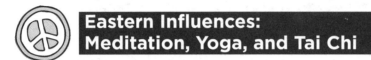

Eastern Influences: Meditation, Yoga, and Tai Chi

Meditation

When you meditate, you focus your attention beyond the normal distractions of life. Meditation allows you to relax and improve your quality of life, and it's simple to do! All you need to meditate is to focus on your breathing.

Let's try meditating right now. After you finish reading this paragraph, close your eyes and breathe deeply from your belly. Count 4 seconds as you slowly inhale and 5 seconds as you exhale. Focus on your breathing and the present moment. There is no right or wrong way to meditate. All states of consciousness are valuable to your meditation practice whether you focus on breathing, sounds, symbols, colors, or positive thoughts. Allow quiet to enter your mind for just 1 or 2 minutes.

Look for everyday opportunities to practice meditation. Try it while walking, standing in line, or while waiting for your computer to boot up. Keep your eyes open and merely focus on your breathing. Or, after a long day, take some time out for an extended period of meditation.

Yoga

Yoga is the practice of stretching and breathing. Yoga brings the mind and body together through mental, physical, and spiritual aspects of the self. It increases energy, endurance, and flexibility; improves blood pressure, sleep, mood, memory, and balance; and reduces stress. Who wouldn't want all of those benefits?

Before you jump into your favorite yoga pose, take some precautions. Certain postures should be avoided if you have high blood pressure, glaucoma, a herniated disc, or a detached retina. Have a conversation with your health-care provider before starting a yoga program.

The best way to learn yoga is to take a basic class or buy a beginner's video. It's generally best to do yoga 1–2 hours after eating or on an empty stomach (which may put you at risk for hypoglycemia). Shoes may not be allowed in yoga studios, so you'll also need to be extra careful with your feet. You should stop a pose if you have pain or find yourself holding your breath. Try any of these:

Chair pose: From a standing position, inhale and extend straightened arms overhead with palms touching. Bend your knees, lower your buttocks, and angle your torso forward slightly (so it looks like you are about to dive into a pool). Hold the pose for three breaths, exhale, and return to a standing position.

Corpse pose: This relaxation pose requires that you lie on your back. Relax your physical, mental, and spiritual being by concentrating on your breathing and intentionally relaxing your muscles from head to toe. Rest in this pose for at least 10 minutes.

Easy pose: A classic meditative pose where you sit with your legs folded, spine straight, and arms relaxed on the knees.

Shoulder stretches: Raise your hands above your head and inhale. Let your hands gently fold behind your head and exhale. Inhale while you touch the base of your neck with your left hand and you grab your left elbow with your right hand. Stretch the shoulder and exhale. Repeat with right arm.

Squat: Stand with feet apart in a wide stance. Bring your palms together in the middle of your chest. Bend your knees and lower your hips down toward your heels. Press your elbows against the inside of your knees. Let your hips lower slightly. Stay in this position for three breaths.

Tai chi

You've probably seen people practicing tai chi in movies or in parks around your city. It looks like a very slow dance. Tai chi can improve your mood, provide relaxation through a meditative state, and build muscle fitness. You can learn tai chi from certified instructors or an instructional video or DVD.

PERSONAL GOAL

Date: _____ I will:

☐ Massage my neck and stretch my shoulders at work.
☐ Stretch when I see my cat or dog stretch.
☐ Find out about local yoga or tai chi classes.
☐ Find a certified tai chi instructor or get a
   "Tai Chi for Diabetes" video from
   www.taichifordiabetes.com.
☐ Make time to meditate for 5 minutes.
☐ Other: _____.

 Will yoga take the
knots out of my stomach?

WEEK
41

 Minute-by-Minute Glucose Monitoring

What is continuous glucose monitoring?

Imagine knowing your blood glucose level minute by minute, hour after hour and being able to "see"—even predict—the direction in which your glucose will be heading in 15 minutes. Well, continuous glucose monitoring (CGM) does just that. It's not perfect (you'll have to double-check highs and lows using a traditional fingerstick test, and most CGM devices require twice-a-day calibration by self–blood glucose monitoring), but it's pretty close. You know what your blood glucose level is just after eating a meal or exercise and have the added security of going to sleep knowing that you will get an alarm *before* your glucose goes too low. These are the benefits that CGM offers.

How does CGM work?

CGM devices display your glucose every 5 minutes. They measure it indirectly by translating the electrical current of the fluid that is just under the skin, called interstitial fluid, into a glucose equivalent value. How? A very small and short needle, called the sensor, is self-inserted through the skin of your abdomen or arm and remains taped in position for a few days. A quarter-size transmitter is snapped into place onto the sensor tape. The transmitter sends a signal with your blood glucose levels to the receiver, a pager-size device that you keep with you. You can see your glucose level on the receiver or, on some models, an insulin pump. CGM devices also have alarms to alert you when your blood glucose is going especially high or low.

Sounds nice, but I bet it's expensive

Yes, *but* a trip to the emergency room, a loss of a day's work, or a disruption in your life spent treating and recovering from hypoglycemia is also quite costly. And for once, you don't need to do the legwork yourself. Talk to your diabetes educator about which CGM is right for you, and they will put you in touch with the company directly, who then will negotiate with your health insurance. Insurance providers often pay the majority of these costs if you are on insulin or have had frequent low blood glucose levels. If you are interested in getting a CGM, ask your health-care provider at your next appointment. Know that it takes a little bit to learn this new system, but it can help you to avoid glucose extremes and time spent in hypoglycemia.

PERSONAL GOAL

Date: _____ I will:

☐ Ask my diabetes care team for a trial CGM I can use before committing to buy one, or how to contact the local CGM representatives to get info on pricing.

☐ Visit these CGM manufacturer websites: DexCom (www.dexcom.com) and Medtronic (www.medtronicdiabetes.com).

☐ Visit a diabetes blog to read what others are saying about CGM.

☐ Check my glucose at a few different times the next 2 days.

☐ Other: _____.

Check, check, check.
CGM is next to OCD in the alphabet.

Over-the-Counter Drugs and Treatments

You can buy many types of medications and treatment remedies without a prescription, but how do you know which ones are safe with your diabetes and other conditions? For instance, some cold medicines may raise your blood glucose, and certain painkillers may raise blood pressure. Here are some tips to think about when buying over-the-counter (OTC) drugs:

- Check the label to know what you're getting. Choose sugar-free products. Search for warnings advising people with diabetes or high blood pressure against taking the medicine or using the product. For example, on wart removal products, you'll see a statement that reads, "Not to be used by people with diabetes."
- Acetaminophen-containing drugs (such as Tylenol) have a risk for severe liver damage *if* more than the maximum recommended dose is taken in 24 hours or if taken by people who have three or more alcoholic drinks in a day.
- Nonsteroidal anti-inflammatory drugs (NSAIDs), such as ibuprofen (Advil), aspirin, naproxen (Aleve), and Ketoprofen, have a risk for stomach bleeding for people more than 60 years old who are taking a blood thinner or steroid, who have three or more alcoholic drinks a day, or who take it longer than directed. NSAIDs are implicated in reducing kidney function (glomelular filtration rate) when used a lot and pose special risk among people with diabetes, especially if proteinuria is present.

Some Diabetes-Friendly OTC Drugs

Allergies	Antacids
Chlor-Trimeton	Alka-Seltzer
Neo-Synephrine	Di-Gel
Claritin	Maalox
Loratadine	Mylanta
	Prilosec
	Tums (sugar-free)
	Zantac

PERSONAL GOAL

Date: _____ I will:

☐ Have a chat with my health-care provider or pharmacist about OTC drugs and treatments that are safe to use.
☐ Bring my vitamins to my registered dietitian for analysis.
☐ Make sure my health-care team knows all of the OTC drugs I take and bring a list of them to every appointment.
☐ Read medication and product labels.
☐ Other: _____.

 I have to buy a magnifying glass to read these warning labels.

The Hospital Twilight Zone

Being hospitalized for a planned or unplanned medical event is like stepping into a *Twilight Zone* episode—it's a new dimension and may be filled with surprises and interesting twists, especially if you let your diabetes guard down.

Ironically, when you're sick in a hospital bed you would think you'd get a break from being your diabetes project manager, but it sometimes doesn't work that way. Some hospitals do not have standardized methods for effectively managing and identifying hyperglycemia, so it's important to keep aware of your diabetes status.

Preparing for the Twilight Zone

You can take several steps to ensure that your hospital stay is as successful as possible. Certainly some hospitals have policies that facilitate self-management of diabetes during your stay.

- Find an advocate or be your own advocate. Ask a family member or friend to watch out for your health while in the hospital or request to see a diabetes educator who can help. Ask your doctor to order blood glucose tests before meals and at bedtime.
- Bring in your meter, supplies, and a complete medication list.
- For planned procedures, try to get the earliest time slot, so you can lower the risks of going low if you have to avoid eating before or after the procedure. Check with your health-care provider about medication and insulin adjustments for the day of the procedure.
- Embrace insulin. Don't freak out if you need insulin during your hospital stay. It is often the best way to maintain good blood glucose levels while you're in the hospital.
- Wear medical identification (bracelet or necklace) in case of

emergencies. This will help emergency staff know that you have diabetes.

- Expect metformin to be stopped during your hospital stay.
- If you wear an insulin pump, call the hospital to find out if it is acceptable to keep using it during your stay and bring all related supplies.

PERSONAL GOAL

Date: _____ I will:

☐ Request to be the first on the list for any procedures or surgery.
☐ Choose an advocate for my hospitalization.
☐ Request to use my own lancets (with the hospital's glucose monitor) to decrease pain.
☐ Ask what medications I am being given and why.
☐ Speak up if my blood glucose levels are not well controlled while I'm in the hospital and ask to speak to the charge nurse, a diabetes educator, or my endocrinologist.
☐ Learn more tips at www.jointcommission.org/ speak_up_diabetes.
☐ Other: _____.

 I used to be afraid of snakes. Now I'm afraid of the hospital.

How high is too high for glucose? There are various degrees of high; in this section, however, we'll cover two conditions that can arise when blood glucose hits dangerously high levels.

What is HHS?

This tongue-twister, hyperosmolar hyperglycemic state, is a rare but serious condition most frequently seen in those who are older and have type 2 diabetes. HHS usually is brought on by something else, such as an illness (pancreatitis, heart attack or stroke, or serious infection) coupled with insulin deficiency and restricted water intake. If left unchecked, it will lead to severe dehydration, seizures, coma, and eventually death. HHS may take days or even weeks to develop, so knowing the warning signs and taking action are critical. Elderly individuals who are unaware of becoming hyperglycemic or are unable to take fluids when necessary (either due to the altered thirst response seen in the elderly or due to being bedridden in a chronic care facility or at a family's home who provide care) are at the highest risk for HHS.

How do I avoid HHS?

That's easy! The best way to avoid HHS is to check your blood glucose levels regularly. That way, if your glucose starts creeping up from 300 to 400 to 500 mg/dL and beyond, you can take action by calling your provider or going to the nearest Emergency Department.

Warning Signs of HHS

- Blood glucose level of more than 600 mg/dL
- Dry, parched mouth
- Extreme thirst (although not always)
- Warm, dry skin that does not sweat
- High fever (over 101°F)
- Sleepiness or confusion
- Loss of vision
- Hallucinations
- Weakness on one side of the body

What is DKA?

Diabetic ketoacidosis (DKA) is a dangerous condition that arises when your body begins burning fat for fuel. This process releases a harmful byproduct called ketones, which can poison the blood. About 5 in 10,000 hospital discharges list DKA as the primary diagnosis, so you hopefully will never experience it. Two-thirds of people who get DKA, however, have type 1 diabetes and 34% have type 2 diabetes. DKA can result in coma and death, so if you see any of the warning signs, get help immediately.

Warning Signs of DKA
- High blood glucose levels
- High levels of ketones in the urine or blood (see below)
- Thirst or a very dry mouth
- Frequent urination

Other symptoms may appear:
- Feeling exhausted
- Dry or flushed skin
- Nausea, vomiting, or abdominal pain (Vomiting can be caused by many illnesses, not just ketoacidosis. If vomiting continues for more than 2 hours, contact your health-care provider.)
- A hard time breathing (short, deep breaths)
- Fruity odor on breath
- A hard time paying attention or confusion

How do I prevent DKA?

DKA can happen during periods of insulin insufficiency, serious infection or extreme stress (trauma, cardiovascular or other emergencies, or surgery), which then can cause significant hyperglycemia. By carefully managing and monitoring your blood glucose levels, and by remembering not to skip doses if you take insulin, you should be able to avoid this critical condition.

How do I test for ketones?

Ketones can be detected in the blood and through the urine. Testing blood is the more precise method for measuring ketones. Urine testing is less reliable but is done easily by dipping a special testing strip of paper into a cup of urine. For people with type 2 diabetes, ketones typically are not checked because it is not a common issue. Your health-care team can recommend whether you need ketone testing as part of your safety net. The supplies needed to check for ketones are more likely to be covered by insurance if you have a prescription.

PERSONAL GOAL

Date: _____ I will:

☐ Ask my health-care provider to go over the signs and symptoms of HHS and DKA.
☐ Promise to check my blood glucose several times a day when I get sick.
☐ Other: _____.

Lower your ketone of voice!

Other Connections to Diabetes

Diabetes has far-reaching effects on many other health issues. Here are a few notable issues not previously covered, listed alphabetically.

Alzheimer's disease

The higher your A1C level (especially when more than 12%), the higher your risk for Alzheimer's disease (AD). Even people with pre-diabetes have a higher risk for AD.

Cancer

Some cancers develop more commonly in people with diabetes (predominantly type 2 diabetes). There is an increased risk for cancers of the liver, pancreas, and endometrium (two fold), as well as for cancers of the colon and rectum, breast, and bladder (up to 1.5-fold). Other cancers (e.g., lung) do not appear to be associated with an increased risk in diabetes, and the evidence for others (e.g., kidney, non-Hodgkin lymphoma) is inconclusive. Confounding issues do exist, like obesity and age, which increase the risk of both cancer and diabetes.

There is one exception: prostate cancer. Several recent studies have shown that diabetes is associated with a lower risk of prostate cancer (search REDEEM for more info). One possible explanation is that diabetes, as well as obesity, lower levels of prostate-specific antigen (PSA) in the blood. High levels of PSA are what prompt biopsies in medical practice, so it is possible that there are simply fewer referrals for biopsies and fewer prostate cancer diagnoses made in this population.

Hearing loss

Diabetes is associated with hearing loss. When is the last time you had a hearing test or a comprehensive examination with an audiologist? What are you doing to prevent hearing loss? Think about that, and turn down the volume on the television and your iPod and minimize your exposure to noisy environments.

Insulin allergies

One of every 200 insulin users may experience an allergic reaction to the additives in the insulin they inject. These additives and buffers help the insulin stay stable and prevent the growth of mold and bacteria. Allergic reactions are quite rare. They tend to appear as redness, itchiness, or hives that remain for several days around injection sites. Allergists can run tests to determine what is causing the reactions and treat your allergy with desensitization, a process that gradually reduces or eliminates a person's allergic reaction to insulin.

Women and lipid management

Women tend to have greater difficulty meeting healthy levels of LDL cholesterol, but they do have better success at meeting HDL cholesterol and triglyceride goals. Type 2 diabetes has clear links to certain types of dyslipidemia (low LDL, high triglycerides, and more small dense LDL particles).

Women with diabetes skip mammogram screening

Despite regular health-care visits, women with diabetes are less likely to get a routine mammogram. It can be easy to put aside other health issues if you're always running to the doctor's office to tend to your diabetes, but mammograms are an important part of female health. Remember to pay attention to the rest of your body.

PERSONAL GOAL

Date: _____ I will:

☐ Enter my weight: _____

☐ Request to see my health-care provider if I'm having a reaction at my insulin injection sites (redness, swelling, itching). The type of insulin may need to be changed, and if that doesn't work, ask about seeing an allergist.

☐ Get my complete cholesterol panel done if I haven't in the past year.

☐ Get my routine mammogram exam.

☐ Ask about cancer risk and screening at my next appointment.

☐ Other: _____.

 Invest in hearing aids—they'll replace all those iPod earphones one day.

Anemia and Diabetes

The connection between diabetes and anemia

Anemia is a condition in which the red blood cells have a reduced ability to carry oxygen throughout the body because they lack a protein called hemoglobin or because their hemoglobin is not working as effectively as it should. Moreover, red blood cells are produced with the help of the kidneys, so if your diabetes affects your kidneys, then anemia may result. Anemia also can be caused by low levels or a lack of iron. People with diabetes have a higher risk for anemia, which can occur in up to 25% of people with the disease.

How do I get tested for anemia?

If there is a chance that you have anemia, you will likely have a blood test called a complete blood count (CBC). The CBC measures your hemoglobin and hematocrit (percentage of red blood cells in blood). If you have low hemoglobin and hematocrit, you may be anemic.

A1C, anemia, and fructosamine

The A1C test measures the amount of glucose stuck to red blood cells. If you have anemia (a common form being sickle cell anemia, but many other types exist), A1C values become unreliable because there are fewer red blood cells to which glucose can attach itself. For people with diabetes and anemia, measuring fructosamine levels is the next best option.

Like A1C, your fructosamine level also represents your average

What Are the Signs of Anemia?

- Feeling tired, weak, or fatigued
- Shortness of breath after very little activity
- Difficulty concentrating
- Frequent headaches
- Pale skin
- Rapid heartbeat
- Chest pain

Did you notice how several of these symptoms are similar to those of hypoglycemia? Take efforts to ensure that you don't have anemia instead of hypoglycemia.

blood glucose level, but only for the previous 2–3 weeks. Fructosamine is formed when protein combines with glucose attached to the inside of a red blood cell. Measuring fructosamine is helpful for people with anemia and for people who have had rapid changes in their diabetes treatment (a new diet or medication).

How can I prevent anemia?

You can prevent anemia in the following ways:
- Protect your kidneys by managing blood glucose and blood pressure levels.
- Get enough iron and vitamins in your diet.
- Determine whether you are at risk for anemia. Although it was mentioned that coffee and tea were fine, if you have any of the symptoms of anemia or are concerned about your risk, consider limiting caffeine as it may interfere with the absorption of iron.

How is anemia treated?

Iron supplements are the common treatment for most forms of anemia (there are many). Don't take iron unless you're told to because extra iron can be rough on your liver. Also, iron makes many people constipated. Some manufacturers solve this issue by combining iron with a stool softener.

For other cases of anemia, there are many different forms of treatment. Some people need regular injections of erythropoietin to tell the kidneys to make more red blood cells. Others need injections of vitamin B12. For life-threatening anemia, people need blood transfusions.

PERSONAL GOAL

Date: _____ I will:

☐ Report any of these symptoms to my health-care provider: feelings of tiredness, weakness, or fatigue; shortness of breath; difficulty concentrating; frequent headaches; pale skin; rapid heartbeat; or chest pain.

☐ Ask to have a fructosamine lab test if I've had a recent change in treatment or if I have anemia (check out the glucose–fructosamine–A1C conversion chart at www.healthyinfo.com/clinical/endo/dm/hga1c.test.shtml).

☐ Learn more about anemia by contacting the National Anemia Action Council at 602-343-7458 or by visiting www.anemia.org.

 Maybe I'm anemic because diabetes causes me to have several irons in the fire.

MONTH 11

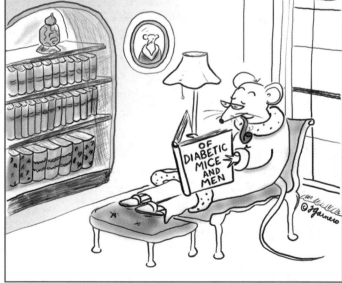

Laughin' Langerhans

By Theresa Garnero

WEEK
44

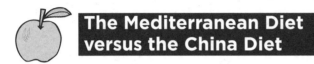

The Mediterranean Diet versus the China Diet

What is the Mediterranean diet? Does it involve a trip to Greece?

Unfortunately, no; when following a Mediterranean diet, the food typically flies to you. The Mediterranean diet has been widely hailed as a more heart-healthy diet than the typical American diet. Rich in fruits, vegetables, fish, bread, potatoes, beans, nuts, and seeds, this diet grew in popularity after a famous research study called the Lyon Diet Heart Study lauded its benefits. Notably, the diet also includes olive oil as an important and "heart healthy" form of monounsaturated fat.

A new study followed 7,500 older adults with diabetes or other heart risks (but initially these individuals did not have heart disease) for 5 years. People on the Mediterranean diet were up to 30% less likely to develop cardiovascular disease than those on the general low-fat diet. It's the blend of Mediterranean diet components, including legumes and fruits as desserts, a wide variety of plant foods, and the quality of fat that promotes heart health; it's not one particular ingredient. It's a combination of what is eaten, and importantly, a combination of what is *not* eaten.

Meet the "China" Diet

A scientist named Colin Campbell who wrote the "China Study" weighed in. He noted that in rural China, there were almost no incidences of coronary disease, which led him to investigate the typical rural Chinese diet. He found that it is practically identical to the Mediterranean diet, with the stark exception of oil. He attributed the higher success of the Chinese diet to the absence of oil, which is prominent in the Mediterranean diet in the form of olive oil.

What Is My Risk for Heart Problems?

In addition to the usual steps to protect your heart with blood pressure, glucose, and cholesterol management via healthy eating, exercise, and medications, a couple of tests give you valuable information about your risk for heart disease.

- **Apo B blood test** (see Day 23). Apo B is more than a measurement of risk (like LDL or non-HDL cholesterol, "non-HDL-C"), it is actually a cause in the progression of artery wall thickening (atherosclerosis).

- **Coronary artery calcium (CAC) scan**. This scan of your heart shows pictures of your coronary arteries and gives you a score that helps you understand your heart attack risk. This is not a routine test. It is expensive, may not be covered by insurance, and may expose you to significant amounts of radiation. The majority of people do not need a CAC scan.

The intent of this section is not to promote obsessive and depressive thinking about health. That doesn't improve the quality of life. It's about knowing your options so you can decide what road to take.

PERSONAL GOAL

Date: _____ I will:

☐ Remove the oil from a meal I cook.

☐ Next time I need a source of protein, I will try reaching for nuts.

☐ Go out to eat in a Chinese restaurant, ask about entrees that use limited or no oil, go easy on the rice, and share the dish to keep portions reasonable.

☐ Have a Greek salad and only use half of the dressing I typically would.

☐ Take the lead of the Mediterranean diet and eat red meat only three times this month.

☐ Other: _____.

 If I go on the Bill Clinton vegan diet, does that make me political?

The Good, the Bad and the Ugly: Menopause and Testosterone

Diabetes aside, hormone imbalances usually are associated with women in menopause. Men also may have hormone issues, however; specifically, they may have low testosterone. This section will help you understand the impact that menopause and low testosterone have on diabetes and your life.

	Menopause	Low testosterone
Description	When menstrual periods stop and ovaries start to shrivel, estrogen and progesterone production fade as well.	Low testosterone levels result from problems in the testes or with the hypothalamus (a small gland in the brain).
Age	Menopause begins around age 51 years, but it can begin as early as 40 years old, or earlier in women whose ovaries are removed surgically.	Low testosterone can begin around age 45 years and older. It affects twice as many men with diabetes as the rest of the population, and only 10% of them get treatment.
Impact on blood glucose levels	May cause fluctuations, especially during perimenopause (the years leading up to menopause).	May raise blood glucose as a result of fatigue, sleep loss, and weight gain.
Symptoms	Menstrual period irregularity (with one to three cycles a year before stopping completely), hot flashes, sweating, irritability, insomnia, and vaginal dryness. Symptoms may continue for years.	Decreased strength and muscle mass, decreased bone density, low sex drive, erectile dysfunction, fatigue, and depression.
Shared diabetes symptoms	Lows: sweating and irritability. Highs: fatigue, mood swings, and vaginal dryness.	Sexual dysfunction, fatigue, and depression.

	Menopause	Low testosterone
Weight	Risk of weight gain.	Overweight men are twice as likely to have low testosterone levels.
Risks	Increased risk for osteoporosis; stress from lack of sleep may raise blood glucose levels.	Increased risk for falls.
Fertility	Fertility decreases after age 40 years, but conception is still possible.	Associated with low sperm count.
Treatment	■ Hormone replacement therapy (HRT) is a treatment that increases hormone levels in women experiencing menopause. ■ The Women's Health Initiative showed that HRT slightly increased the risks of breast cancer, stroke, and dementia. Specific study findings for the estrogen-plus-progesterone group compared with the placebo group were numerous, and the trial was stopped due to increased breast cancer risk and lack of overall benefit (a 41% increase in strokes, a 29% increase in heart attacks, a doubling of rates of venous thromboembolism [blood clots], a 22% increase in total cardiovascular disease, a 26% increase in breast cancer, a 37% reduction in cases of colorectal cancer, a 33% reduction in hip fracture rates, a 24% reduction in total fractures, and no difference in total, all-cause mortality rates). ■ HRT prevents osteoporosis. ■ Prescription vaginal estrogen (in cream, tablet, or ring formats) may help with pain and lubrication issues. OTC vaginal moisturizers are also available.	The primary method of treatment is to increase testosterone levels by adding more. This is achieved in a few ways: ■ Gels that can be applied to the stomach or upper arms. ■ Patches that can be applied once a week. ■ Injections that are given about every 2 weeks.

PERSONAL GOAL

Date: _____ I will:

☐ Consult with my health-care team about the best approach to deal with my hormone issues.
☐ Contact the North American Menopause Society at 440-442-7550 or visit www.menopause.org.
☐ Ask to be tested for low testosterone and have the blood test in the morning, when levels are peaking.
☐ Report breast tenderness to my health-care team.
☐ Report my decreased strength or height to my health-care provider.
☐ Other: _____.

My glands have issues.

Caring for Your Sweetie, *and* Yourself!

Are you part of the support network for someone with diabetes? Who fills that role for you? A partner, parent, sibling, or friend? You both probably experience some similar emotional reactions to diabetes, such as frustration, anger, resentment, or fear. It's a tricky balance. It's like being in the passenger seat of a moving car: the person with diabetes or other health condition is the driver, and the passenger is implicated in the outcomes and wants to help, but no one likes an obtrusive back-seat driver.

This means you must learn how to communicate your needs. How can you be helpful or get the right kind of support without neglecting your own well-being? You and your loved one need to learn some skills akin to tightrope walking on this life journey together. Each person needs to remember his or her role and support—not dictate—how the self-care can happen. This includes agreeing on strategies of when and how to ask for help. For example, it can be tempting to have foods in the house that you know will be too good to pass up. If the person without diabetes insists on eating these foods, and you can't avoid eating them, then you have a problem! You can negotiate and meet somewhere in the middle. With a little practice and a lot of patience, you'll find out what works.

PERSONAL GOAL

Date: _____ I will:

☐ Talk to a friend about the stress I experience as a caregiver.
☐ Read and share the caregiver etiquette guide from the Behavioral Diabetes Institute (www.behavioraldiabetesinstitute.org/downloads/Etiquette-Card.pdf#zoom=100).
☐ Invite my loved one to make similar diet changes.
☐ Make a healthy home-cooked meal for my loved one. Remember the flowers.
☐ Other: _____.

WEEK 46

Going the Extra Mile

This section is for those of you who are going the extra mile with an activity program, or for those of you who are flat-out athletes.

Exercise Nutrition

When your body is at rest, it gets about 60% of its energy from fat and 40% from carbohydrates. During exercise, the body turns to carbohydrates for energy. The harder the workout and intensity, the more the body leans on carbs for fuel. If you are exercising before or between meals, you may need a snack, especially if you plan on more than 30 minutes of activity.

As a review, consider having a snack before exercise to prevent hypoglycemia if your blood glucose is less than 100 mg/dL, you're going to exercise before a meal, you will be active for more than an hour, or your medication or insulin is peaking. Based on a 150-pound person, you'd need about 30–40 grams of carbohydrate for 1 hour of moderate-intensity exercise or as much as 55 grams for high-intensity workouts. If you weigh more, you'll need a bigger snack. In addition, the protein requirements for athletes dedicated to

Quick Snacks to Help Fuel My Body

- Sports drinks with up to 8% carbohydrate (higher percentages may cause cramping and diarrhea).
- Electrolytes for events more than 2 hours in length.
- GU Energy Gel (it's maltodextrin and fructose) or GU Sports Drink (call 510-527-4664 or visit www.guenergy.com to find out more).
- Don't forget water. You need it to prevent dehydration. Have some before your workout, when you start to sweat, and as needed to replenish after your workout.

their sport are nearly double (about 100 grams a day). Remember to discuss exercise nutrition with a dietitian before becoming a full-time athlete.

How do I get my body ready for a several-hour event?

Eat a high-carb diet for about a week before the event, which is about 4 grams of carb per pound of body weight. For someone who weighs 150 pounds, that's 600 grams of carb a day. Make sure your medication can cover the added carbs so you won't be running on high blood glucose levels. Be sure to taper down your activity a couple of days before the big event. Your body needs a couple of days to rebuild nutrient stores and repair tissue. If you are trying to run a marathon, participate in a triathlon, or do something equally ambitious and you haven't seen your dietitian for an individualized nutrition plan, I will come and find you. That's flat-out dangerous. Make exercise nutrition a part of your training program.

Glucose Chutes and Ladders

Strenuous exercise can whip your blood glucose levels around like a birthday balloon in the wind. Let's review some key points.

- Hypoglycemia may occur during the exercise or be delayed into the next day. Frequently check your glucose before, during, and up to 24 hours after exercise.
- Hyperglycemia may result temporarily from bursting-type or competitive sports, such as weightlifting, baseball, track, swimming, gymnastics, and figure skating. This is caused from a release of hormones that free stored glucose during exercise.

Insulin Deep Thoughts

On the days you exercise hard, you will need a different plan for your insulin doses. Consider some basic principles, but remember to talk to your health-care provider before you make changes.

Basal insulin

Unless you are planning to exercise for more than 2 hours, your long-acting insulin dose can stay the same. For more than 2 hours of activity, plan on reducing your basal dose by 20% (up to 30% for hard-core, several-hour events) for the day before the event. Be aware that extreme temperatures can affect your blood glucose levels.

Bolus insulin

You may want to take 70% of your usual premeal insulin dose for 30–60 minutes of activity, 50% for 1 hour of heavy-duty exercise, or 35% for more than 2 hours of vigorous exercise.

Correction doses

Use half of what you normally would to cover your highs.

PERSONAL GOAL

Date: _____ I will:

☐ Pay a visit to a registered dietitian who is also a CDE and specializes in exercise (call the American Association of Diabetes Educators at 800-338-3633 and ask for help locating someone from the Physical Activity Communities of Interest).

☐ Talk to my health-care provider about adjusting my medications to handle extra carbs during periods of extreme activity.

☐ Check my blood glucose every 30–60 minutes during vigorous exercise, more often if I feel strange.

☐ Carry my hypoglycemia treatment pack and ketone test strips.

☐ Other: _____.

 Sugar Ray had to live up to his name.

It's that time, again?

Have you had your eyes checked recently? A dilated eye exam is recommended within a few months after being diagnosed with type 2 diabetes and then every year, regardless of how long you've had diabetes. You may need more frequent exams if you have a condition that requires monitoring. Women with diabetes who are planning a pregnancy also should have a dilated eye exam.

Skipping your regular eye checkups can put you at risk of serious eye complications, the most serious of which can be prevented—blindness.

What are some common eye problems related to diabetes?

Some of the common eye problems related to diabetes are as follows:

- *Blurry vision.* High blood glucose levels may cause blurry vision, which can go away after blood glucose levels return to the target range, providing they haven't been high for years.
- *Cataracts.* A clouding of the lens is twice as likely to happen in people with diabetes and at a younger age than in those without diabetes. Cataracts can be removed surgically.
- *Glaucoma.* A condition in which increased pressure in the eye damages the optic nerve (the main nerve in the eye) over a long time. The first symptom of glaucoma is reduced vision out of the corners of the eyes. Glaucoma can be treated with medications or surgery. If left untreated, glaucoma can lead to blindness.
- *Retinopathy.* The most common eye problem associated with diabetes is retinopathy, in which the tiny blood vessels leak fluid into the light-sensing lining in the back of the eye (called the retina). This can lead to vision loss. In the early stage, it's called background retinopathy and typically no symptoms are present. In the advanced stage, proliferative retinopathy can develop, in which the eye grows new blood vessels that are fragile, tend to grow in the wrong places, and bleed into

the eyeball. If left untreated, this can lead to blindness. With timely treatment, blindness often can be prevented. You can protect your sight by having yearly checkups with an ophthalmologist.

What are the treatments for retinopathy and macular edema?

For those with advanced retinopathy and significant macular edema, laser surgery is a common and effective way to treat it. Why laser? It is used to zap the leaking blood vessels, which stops the bleeding and keeps the oxygen flowing to the healthy vessels. Not all retinopathy needs laser surgery. For diabetic macular edema, an injection of anti-vascular endothelial growth factor (anti-VEGF) is a standard treatment. You can protect your sight by having yearly checkups with an ophthalmologist or optometrist so you can catch any possible issues early on.

My vision isn't great: What's out there to help?

Many resources can assist you if you are living with visual impairment. To begin with, every state has low-vision and blindness agencies that are dedicated to helping you maintain your independence. Specialists can determine the best lighting and magnification products to meet your needs. These include handheld devices, bifocals, large-print reading materials, and computer screen programs that automatically can increase the font size or even describe everything displayed on the screen.

Your diabetes care team can help you get low-vision equipment for diabetes self-management. For example, talking blood glucose meters are available. In addition, manufacturers make syringe magnifiers, needle guides, and vial stabilizers for those who have trouble seeing. Technology can help you learn new ways to stay healthy with diabetes when you have visual impairment. Even though you may never need these additional resources, you may know someone who could benefit:

- The National Federation of the Blind (410-659-9314; www.nfb.org). Enter "living with blindness and diabetes" in search field.
- The American Council of the Blind (800-424-8666; www.acb.org). Of.fers a free monthly publication, *The Braille Forum.*
- The American Foundation for the Blind (800-232-5463; www.afb.org).

- The National Library Service for the Blind and Physically Handicapped (202-707-5100; www.loc.gov/nls). Offers a Postage-free Talking Book Program with audiobooks and the equipment to play the tapes; texts in Braille.

PERSONAL GOAL

Date: _____ I will:

☐ Make an appointment to see an eye doctor; your eyes will love you for it.
☐ Ask my pharmacist or CDE about magnifying devices.
☐ Make a date to quit smoking.
☐ Avoid secondhand smoke.
☐ Talk with my doctor about my blood pressure.
☐ Other: _____.

Seek Out Joy

Having diabetes requires much effort and energy. You've had to focus your daily attention on health matters. It is difficult to find the balance; turn off the constant thinking. Look for reasons to smile or feel good. Here are some examples:

- A hot shower when you're freezing.
- Geese flying overhead in a perfect "V" formation.
- Microwave popcorn.
- Food delivered to your door.
- Your suitcase being the first at the baggage carousel.

PERSONAL GOAL

Date: _____ I will:

☐ Turn off the television, close my eyes for 5 minutes, and let my thoughts drift.

☐ Buy a bouquet (or pick one from my garden) and marvel at the colors of nature.

☐ Be a source of love.

☐ Slow down a little bit to stay "in the moment."

☐ Call a friend who is upbeat.

☐ Pick up that book I've been meaning to read.

☐ Let go of something that I've been resenting.

☐ Other: _____.

 I heard Karma means watching your body, mouth, and mind. You're fun to watch.

MONTH 12

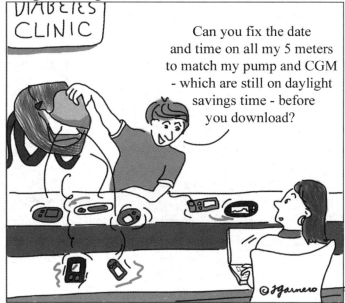

Laughin' Langerhans   By Theresa Garnero

WEEK
48

Pause for Podiatry

Diabetes puts you at a risk for foot problems. You can keep your feet pristine with glucose and blood pressure control, good foot care, early detection of foot problems, and regular foot exams. Now, get ready for a lot of "ifs": If blood glucose levels are high for months on end, the nerves going to your feet can lose their ability to detect pain, heat, cold, and pressure. If you can't feel in your feet and get a cut, blister, or callus, you may not know it. If you have circulation problems, healing becomes difficult, and if your blood glucose level is elevated, bacteria will thrive. Even a small break in the skin can turn into a terrible infection under these circumstances.

Do I need to see the podiatrist if I'm not having problems?

No, but you do need a comprehensive foot exam by your medical provider and to establish a podiatrist in the event you ever need specialized services. A podiatrist will check the sensitivity of your feet with a monofilament (a harmless piece of plastic) and a tuning fork. You also may have a Doppler test (a painless in-office ultrasound) screening for peripheral arterial disease (PAD) and X-rays to check for bone problems. Your podiatrist can trim your nails to prevent them from becoming ingrown, thin down thick nails, and provide custom footwear (orthotics) designed to reduce pressure and foot pain.

Do Any of These Apply to You?

If any of the following apply to you, then you should make an appointment with a podiatrist as soon as possible.

- Do you have an open wound? (Get to the doctor today. It can save a limb.)
- Do you have a corn, blister, or callus?
- Are there any red spots on your foot?
- Do your feet have a strong odor?
- Are your feet cold most of the time?
- Are you able to cut your own toenails?
- Are your toenails thick, jagged, or ingrown?
- Is the skin between your toes cracked?
- Do you have deep cracks in the skin of your feet?
- Do you have numbness, tingling, or pain?
- Do your feet kill you at the end of the day or keep you up at night?
- Is one of your feet hot and the other not?

PERSONAL GOAL

Date: _____ I will:

☐ Check the bottom of my feet daily (use a mirror if needed).
☐ Put lotion on my heels daily.
☐ Find a podiatrist by calling my insurance to see who is covered, or check the American Podiatric Medical Association for local podiatrists at www.apma.org (301-581-9200).
☐ Get a PAD screening test if I'm more than 50 years old or have leg pain or cramping.
☐ Avoid exposure to smoke.
☐ Other: _____

My little toe has a corn, and my big one has a cauliflower.

Ready, Set...Stop?

Are you having difficulty sticking to an exercise program? Nearly half of people who start an activity regimen stop within 6 months. For many people, a great motivator is to join a gym or health club. Some people swear by them, others just swear.

Gyms and Health Clubs: Tips for the Savvy Shopper

1. **Convenience.** If the gym is more than 12 minutes away, people tend to stop going. Pick one close by.
2. **Timing.** Stop by to see how busy it is at the time you plan to exercise to see if enough equipment is available. Peak times are typically 4–7 p.m.
3. **Equipment.** Check for a variety of well-maintained machines. If you see dust bunnies and built-up grime, go elsewhere.
4. **Personal trainers and class variety.** Ask about classes and fitness professionals who can help you with an individualized program.
5. **Trial memberships.** Most gyms offer a free daily or weekly pass. Give it a test drive. Do you like the environment? Does it make you want to return?
6. **Get recommendations.** Ask someone who belongs to the gym what they like and dislike.
7. **Expense.** Ask what's included in your contract or if there are hidden fees (sometimes towels and lockers cost extra). Ask about special offers or if the gym is part of a chain, so you can go to different locations. Ask whether their policy allows you to suspend your membership for illness and vacation and whether penalties apply if you cancel your membership.

PERSONAL GOAL

Date: _____ I will:

☐ Ponder what it will take to become active the rest of my life.

☐ Research some local gyms and visit one.

☐ Other: _____.

My active voice works out every day. Now I need to get my body to listen.

WEEK
49

While You Weren't Sleeping

A good night's sleep seems to be on the verge of extinction. Short-changing sleep causes more than a droopy-eyed look of confusion and midday yawn-a-thons—it raises blood glucose levels, causes other medical issues, and shortens your life.

Why is sleep important?

Every organ depends on adequate sleep to function properly. Sleep is a dynamic, complex activity. Lack of sleep interferes with your ability to produce insulin and fight illness and increases your risk for high blood pressure, depression, heart attacks, and strokes. If that's not bad enough, inadequate sleep increases stress hormones, causing the body to store fat and making it more difficult to lose weight.

What Is Sleep Apnea?

Sleep apnea is a sleeping disorder in which you stop breathing for periods of up to 1 minute, and it may occur hundreds of times a night. Sleep apnea is common with type 2 diabetes, with men, and with individuals who are overweight, smoke, or drink too much alcohol. It can increase glucose and blood pressure as well as the risk for cardiovascular disease, stroke, and death. Signs of sleep apnea include loud snoring, headaches, dry mouth, feeling exhausted upon awakening, and sleeping at inappropriate times during the day. A sleep specialist can diagnose the problem through physical exams, a trip to a sleep clinic, or by home sleep testing equipment. Treatment options include using a continuous positive airway pressure (CPAP) device to keep the airway open during sleep (although wearing this mask is difficult for many), dental appliances to keep the tongue from falling to the back of the throat, and surgical procedures.

How Can I Get More Sleep?

Sleep hygiene

The bed is meant for sleep and sex, and if you're missing one, check out this list for sleep hygiene recommendations.

- Put yourself on a timeout to wind down for 30 minutes before bed.
- Get a new mattress or pillow.
- Try to go to bed and wake up around the same time every day.
- Avoid exercise and eating right before bed.
- Avoid caffeine (coffee or drinks) after lunch.
- Limit liquids after dinner.
- Limit alcohol intake.
- Don't eat or watch television in bed.
- Try relaxing breathing exercises when you get into bed.
- After an *estimated* 20–30 minutes of not falling asleep, get out of bed (and don't obsessively watch the clock or it can stress you out and wake you up). Then, do something relaxing, like listening to music or reading something light, until you are sleepy enough to return to bed. Don't set up camp on the couch or you'll begin to associate sleep with the couch and not your bed.
- Talk to your health-care provider.

Medications

Less than 10% of people with sleep disturbances take medication for the condition. If you need help sleeping, these can improve your quality of life on a short-term basis. Be careful not to use them long term as they have side effects and be sure to report any weird symptoms. After taking sleeping pills for more than a few weeks, rare side effects may occur. Best to learn other ways to get your sleep through the listed sleep hygiene techniques as well as to learn how to deal with the stress that is in your life.

PERSONAL GOAL

Date: _____ I will:

☐ Avoid stimulating or upsetting activities before bed (e.g., news, bills, hot topics with my spouse).
☐ Write down my to-do list before my head hits the pillow.
☐ Set the thermostat to 68–72°F.
☐ Keep my bedroom dark during sleep (e.g., wear an eyeshade or use blackout shades, clips to hold curtains in place, 45-watt light bulbs).
☐ Within an hour of waking, find natural sunlight to help wake me up.
☐ Note hours slept in my blood glucose logbook.
☐ Find a local sleep center at www.sleepcenters.org.
☐ Reduce clutter.
☐ Other: _____.

 I tried counting sheep.
They ran off thinking I was a zombie.

What's the Alternative?

Complementary or alternative medicine may be helpful as a holistic approach to diabetes self-management. Mention any therapies you use to your health-care team, so they have the complete picture and can advise you about potential safety issues.

What about dietary supplements?

Nearly half of U.S. adults use dietary supplements, ranging from a daily multivitamin to fish oil pills. Why? Most people believe it will improve their health. The American Diabetes Association does not recommend these as standard therapies, however, as the effects may be small and they are not without side effects. It's best to consult an RD or your primary care provider about their safety because many supplements can have negative effects when combined with prescription medication.

To present validated research, the following tables include a review of common dietary supplements specific to diabetes and related conditions. The review was conducted via Natural Standard, whose tagline is "The Authority on Integrative Medicine" (access to this information typically is available to professionals at major health-care institutions). Natural Standard uses a grading scale to reflect the level of available evidence in support of a given therapy's effectiveness. Expert opinion and "folkloric precedent" are not included in this assessment. The thorough database even translates international research journals.

Each therapy or supplement receives a grade pertaining to evidence of its benefit (A through F, terms we can identify with from school days!); evidence of harm is noted in their summaries. Only common supplements with a grade A, B, or C are listed.

Forms of Complementary and Alternative Medicine

- Acupuncture
- Ayurveda
- Biofeedback
- Chelation
- Chiropractic
- Energy healing
- Herbal remedies and dietary supplements
- Homeopathy
- Hypnosis
- Massage
- Naturopathy
- Reiki therapy

Level of evidence "grade"	Criteria
A (strong scientific evidence)	Statistically significant evidence of benefit from more than two properly randomized controlled trials (RCTs), OR evidence from one properly conducted RCT AND one properly conducted meta-analysis, OR evidence from multiple RCTs with a clear majority of the properly conducted trials showing statistically significant evidence of benefit AND with supporting evidence in basic science, animal studies, or theory.
B (good scientific evidence)	Statistically significant evidence of benefit from one or two properly randomized trials, OR evidence of benefit from more than one properly conducted meta-analysis OR evidence of benefit from more than one cohort, case-control, nonrandomized trial AND with supporting evidence in basic science, animal studies, or theory. This grade applies to situations in which a well-designed RCT reports negative results but stands in contrast to the positive efficacy results of multiple other less-well-designed trials or a well-designed meta-analysis, while awaiting confirmatory evidence from an additional well-designed RCT.
C (unclear or conflicting scientific evidence)	Evidence of benefit from more than one small RCT(s) without adequate size, power, statistical significance, or quality of design by objective criteria, OR conflicting evidence from multiple RCTs without a clear majority of the properly conducted trials showing evidence of benefit or ineffectiveness, OR evidence of benefit from more than one cohort, case-control, nonrandomized trial AND without supporting evidence in basic science, animal studies, or theory, OR evidence of efficacy only from basic science, animal studies, or theory.

Name (grade)	Possible effects	Considerations
Alpha-lipoic acid (A)	Increases insulin sensitivity, helps treat nerve pain (neuropathy).	Can cause hypoglycemia with insulin or pills that cause insulin release. Use cautiously with thyroid problems.
Beta-glucan (B)	In several randomized studies, oat bran diets, barley, and barley products enriched with beta-glucan positively affected postprandial blood glucose, postprandial endothelial function, and insulin in patients with type 2 diabetes	Use cautiously in patients with diabetes or in those taking antidiabetic agents, as based on human and animal study, beta-glucan may alter blood glucose levels.

Name (grade)	Possible effects	Considerations
Bitter melon (C)	May lower glucose (studies were poorly designed) and if taken with cholesterol med, lower Apo B.	Risk of hypoglycemia.
Chromium picolinate (C)	May improve insulin sensitivity and glucose control.	May pose an increased risk of hypoglycemia and renal problems.
Cinnamon (C)	Increases insulin sensitivity. May lower total cholesterol and TG levels and increase HDL levels.	May cause hypoglycemia when combined with other diabetes drugs. Use cautiously with anticoagulants.
Fenugreek (C)	May improve blood glucose levels. May improve cholesterol levels when taken with a cholesterol med.	Don't use during pregnancy due to miscarriage risk. Risk of low potassium (hypokalemia) when taken with antiarrhythmic agents and some diuretics. Can have hypothyroid effect.
Garlic (C)	May improve blood glucose levels; increases insulin production and glucose storage in the liver.	Has anticlotting effects and may decrease the effectiveness of other drugs.
Ginseng (American or Asian types) (B)	May improve blood glucose levels; may prevent progression of kidney damage.	May increase blood pressure and cause insomnia. Risk of bleeding when used with anticoagulant. May increase risk for irregular heartbeat.
Grape seed extract (B)	May halt the progression of retinopathy or improve vision in healthy individuals. May lower LDL in combination with chromium.	Use cautiously with blood pressure or bleeding disorders (especially if taking an ACE inhibitor or anticoagulant).
Gymnema (B)	May improve blood glucose levels for type 1 and 2 diabetes. If used with a cholesterol med, may lower total cholesterol, TG, and LDL.	May cause hypoglycemia.
Konjac gluco-mannan (A)	May decrease fasting and after meal glucose.	May cause hypoglycemia (it can decrease intestinal absorption of sulfonylureas and other drugs) and low blood pressure. Use cautiously with thyroid problems.
Magne-sium (B)	Improves insulin sensitivity and action.	May cause diarrhea; avoid if you have kidney problems. May cause hypoglycemia.

Name (grade)	Possible effects	Considerations
Nopal (prickly pear) (B)	Improves blood glucose levels and insulin sensitivity.	Risk of hypoglycemia. Use cautiously with thyroid problems.
Omega-3 fatty acids (fish oil) (A)	Improves triglycerides; decreases risk for stroke and heart attack.	May increase blood glucose levels.
Policosa-nol (B)(C)	Improves cholesterol levels. B for coronary heart disease; C for cholesterol.	Use cautiously with anticlotting medications (like aspirin).
Psyllium (C)	Slows absorption of glucose and fat.	Reduces absorption of other drugs; risk of hypoglycemia.
Whey pro-tein (B)	May lower after-meal glucose (by increasing glucagon-like peptide-1); may lower total cholesterol, LDL and TG levels.	Risk of hypoglycemia. Use cautiously if taking blood pressure medications. Avoid if allergic to milk.
Vitamins (multi-vitamins contain 3 or more vitamins, such as vitamins A, B, and C, or more and min-erals)	Multivitamins can help people obtain recommended intakes of vitamins and minerals when they cannot meet these needs from food alone. Keep in mind that many people with diabetes do not get enough vitamin D. You may need to take more vitamin D3 than a multivitamin offers.	

Better safe than sorry

Supplement manufacturers are not regulated in the same fashion as drug companies, and they don't even have to register their products. Look for the U.S. Pharmacopeia (USP) label on supplements; it guarantees the integrity (content and dosage) of the supplement. Supplements aren't substitutes for healthy eating and being active.

What about probiotics?

Probiotics are live microorganisms that have a health benefit, especially for people with diabetes, and also may help with weight management. They are sold as conventional foods and as dietary supplements. Most probiotics are *Lactobacillus* or *Bifidobacterium* species, but *Saccharomyces* (a yeast) and *S. thermophilus* (a yogurt starter culture) are also common. Some (but not all) dairy products contain live, active cultures with added potential health effects. Talk with your health-care provider to find out the best one. A consumer resource guide is available at www.isapp.net/docs/Consumer_Guidelines-probiotic.pdf.

PERSONAL GOAL

Date: _____ I will:

☐ Consult a health practitioner trained in the use of supplements (e.g., a registered dietitian, pharmacist).

☐ Tell my health-care team about all the supplements I'm taking.

☐ Take one multivitamin with breakfast.

☐ Stay away from scam products that say that you can permanently lose weight without exercising or that block the absorption of fat or carbohydrates.

☐ Visit the National Center for Complementary and Alternative Medicine of the National Institutes of Health (a free resource that provides referenced clinical information) at www.nccam.nih.gov.

☐ Other: _____ .

 Can I use those herbal supplements as salad garnish?

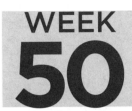

 Sequence for Success

You can monitor your own diabetes track record by using this form. Work with your diabetes care team to cover each of these standards of care. Find a provider who matches or understands your style of communication.

Every visit	Date ____	Date ____	Date ____	Date ____	Goals* or notes
Blood pressure					Below 140/80 mmHg
Weight					
Glucose review					Before meals 70–130 mg/dL; 2 hours after meals less than 180 mg/dL
Medication review					
Meal review					
Activity review					

Every visit	Date ____	Date ____	Date ____	Date ____	Goals* or notes
Foot inspection					
Voice your concerns					

Every 3–6 months	Date ____	Date ____	Date ____	Date ____	Goals*
A1C					Below 7%

Every 6 months	Date ____		Date ____		Goals*
Dentist					Cleaning and checkup
Check disaster kit					Renew and replenish

Yearly	Date(s) _____	Goals* or notes
Physical exam		
Complete cholesterol panel		HDL: more than 40 mg/dL for men; more than 50 for women LDL: less than 100 mg/dL (less than 70 is best) Triglycerides: less than 150 mg/dL (less than 100 is best)
Diabetes educator		
Eye exam		
Foot exam		
Flu shot		
Urine albumin		less than 30 mg/dL (kidney test)

Ask about the pneumonia vaccine, aspirin use, hepatitis B, and a thyroid checkup.

*Goals are those suggested by the American Diabetes Association. Your health-care provider may recommend different goals and frequency of tests and visits.

PERSONAL GOAL

Date: _____ I will:

☐ Make sure that I'm getting all of these tests done (and won't assume that it's "okay" if I don't hear anything).

☐ Bring the chart to my appointments and ask them to enter my results.

☐ Ask my health-care provider to conduct tests and evaluations that he or she may have forgotten.

☐ Other: _____.

All this performance review for my health care and I don't even get a raise?!

Diabetes Burnout

How are you feeling about having diabetes about now? Are you keeping up or fed up with self-care? Diabetes burnout is a common phenomenon when dealing with the never-ending demands of managing diabetes. Do you ever feel . . .

- Aggravated?
- Angry?
- Like you explode easily at seemingly unimportant things?
- Beat up by diabetes?
- Bothered by everything related to your diabetes?
- Deprived of your favorite foods?
- Like no one understands your struggle?
- Negative and irritable?
- Overwhelmed?
- Exhausted?
- Hopeless?
- Isolated?
- Like there is a lack of support from those closest to you?

Have you stopped regularly checking your blood glucose, missed medical appointments, skipped refilling a prescription, or reverted to your old ways of eating that weren't in the best interest of your health? All of these are common, including the feelings described in the previous list, and indicate that you may be experiencing diabetes burnout.

Dodging the Blood Glucose Police

Do your family and friends help or hinder your efforts? Statements like the following don't help you or anyone else with diabetes:

- "You really shouldn't eat that." (But he or she keeps sweets in the house.)
- "You seem mad. Is your blood glucose high again?"
- "Why can't you just get your blood glucose under control?"
- "Why don't you exercise and lose weight?" (But he or she won't join you for a walk or any activity.)
- "Your doctor's not going to be happy with you." (But he or she brings home foods that aren't going to help your diabetes.)

If you feel like your support group is not so supportive, speak up. Point out that by being the blood glucose police, they're not helping you. Tell them that you're doing your best and that you need a cheerleader in your corner, not a traffic cop writing you tickets every time you slip up.

Diabetes burnout puts people at greater risk of future complications and big problems in the present, like severe highs and lows.

If you're feeling discouraged or overwhelmed, seek out help from your health-care team and support team right away. Many people feel down about diabetes, so there's no shame in bringing it up.

PERSONAL GOAL

Date: _____ I will:

☐ Say "no" to things that don't support my goals, including people.
☐ Identify what's stressing me out.
☐ Get my diabetes care team involved if I think I'm experiencing diabetes burnout.
☐ Strive for my best and avoid perfectionism.
☐ Work on a hobby.
☐ Read a poem, look at art, or feed the birds.
☐ Other: _____.

 Have a plan B, plan C, and plan Hawaii!

WEEK
51

Panorama Point

Things don't always happen as planned, yet they have a way of working out. Getting diagnosed with diabetes may have been quite a shock and sent your life in a new direction. You may long for the life you had before getting diagnosed with diabetes, but you are still the same person, only wiser and potentially healthier because you're now invested in your mental and physical well-being.

As with any crisis, your diabetes diagnosis has presented you with an opportunity to reflect and regroup. Looking back, what do you see from this vantage point? What have you learned about diabetes, yourself, and those around you? What strengths and vulnerabilities have you discovered?

Before we part, let's take some time to review your journey so far. This is not the end. It's the beginning. Another chapter in your life is about to unfold. Remember to be strong and resourceful as you continue on. Even with diabetes, life still can have passion—so enjoy yourself. And remember to find reasons to smile.

YEAR IN REVIEW

Date: _____

Look back over this past year and review the goals you made for yourself, focusing on one key decision at a time. Next to each area in the following table, jot down at least one successful change you've made and one area that could use attention.

Keys to success	Successful change	Needs attention
Eat wisely		
Be active		
Check numbers		
Reduce stress		
Understand medications		
Solve Problems		
Reduce risks		
Add humor		

Having some trouble?

Here are some things to think about as you fill out the chart.

- On average, are my blood glucose levels 70–130 mg/dL before meals and less than 180 mg/dL 2 hours after meals?
- Can I sometimes identify why my blood glucose levels fluctuate?
- Was my last A1C less than 7%?
- Is my blood pressure less than 140/80 mmHg?
- Is my LDL cholesterol less than 100 mg/dL? (Or, if you are on maximal tolerated statin therapy, is your LDL 30–40% lower than your initial baseline?)
- Is my diet diabetes friendly?
- Am I getting regular physical activity?
- Have I forgotten to take my medication this past week?
- Do I sabotage or rescue myself?
- Have I laughed at myself lately?
- Are my thoughts more positive than negative?
- Do I plan ahead to deal with potential problems?
- Am I willing to ask for help?
- Do I report problems?
- Have I replaced my toothbrush recently?

PERSONAL GOAL

Thumb through this book on a regular basis so you can choose new goals or revisit ones you've already selected. In addition, here are some new ideas.

Date: _____ I will:

☐ Go to a spa.
☐ Decide what I am *not* going to eat today.
☐ Find an activity that I love to do.
☐ Embrace slow, lasting weight loss by focusing on getting strong and healthy.
☐ Attend an intensive diabetes program.
☐ Research and investigate the latest in diabetes breakthroughs.
☐ Participate in a diabetes study, so I can help improve the status for all people with diabetes.
☐ Get involved with or volunteer for a diabetes organization in my community.

 Health is a form of art. Look at it twice and you see something else: a new color, feeling, or perspective. Blessings, as you build your masterpiece that is you!

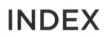

INDEX

Note: Page numbers followed by an *f* refer to figures. Page numbers followed by a *t* refer to tables.

A

A1C (glycosylated hemoglobin), 12–13, 15, 156, 294, 297–298. *See also* estimated average glucose
Academy of Nutrition and Dietetics, 209
acetaminophen-containing drugs, 287
activity. *See also* exercise
  athlete, 308–310
  benefit, 20–22
  blood glucose level, 131
  blood pressure health, 83
  calorie burning, 177–178
  diary, 37*f*
  inspiring, 155
  prediabetes, 11
  preparing for, 44–47
  standards, 106–108
  walking, 79–81
adolescent, 106
adult, 106, 185
advocate, 165–166, 289
aerobic activity, 107
African American population, 83, 114, 161*t*, 185
African American/Pan-African celebration, 240
airport security screening, 175
albuminuria, 44
alcohol, 76–77, 83, 86, 110, 142, 191, 238, 240, 320
allergy, 287, 295
alpha-blocker, 160*t*
alpha-glucosidase inhibitor, 55*t*
alpha-lipoic acid, 323*t*
alternative medicine, 322–326
alternative site testing, 241, 274–275
Alzheimer's disease (AD), 294
American Association of Diabetes Educators, 24, 208, 310
American Council of the Blind, 312
American Council on Exercise, 254

American Dental Association's Seal of Acceptance, 273
American Diabetes Association (ADA), 21, 24, 68, 103, 164, 208, 240, 322
American Diabetes Association Recognized Education Program, 24
American Diabetes Association's 2013 Standards of Care, 80, 225
American Foundation for the Blind, 313
American Heart Association, 82
Amish people, 79
amphetamine, 264
amputation, 45
amylin, 268
amylinomimetic, 57*t*, 268
anemia, 13, 116, 241, 297–299
anger, 120
angina, 230
angiotensin II receptor blockers (ARBs), 159*t*–161*t*
angiotensin-converting enzyme (ACE) inhibitors, 159*t*–161*t*
ankle reflex, 257
antacid, 287
antiplaque–anti-gingivitis toothpaste, 119
antiseptic mouthwash, 119
anti-vascular endothelial growth factor (anti-VEGF) therapy, 312
Apo B blood test, 303
apolipoprotein B (Apo B), 104
apps, 233
Armchair Fitness videos, 272
arthritis, 270
artificial sweeteners, 18*t*, 126
Asian American population, 114
aspirin, 231
atherosclerosis, 230, 303
athlete, 151, 308–310
autoimmune disease, 252–253

B

bagel, 112
bariatric surgery, 249–250
Barnard, Neal, 62
bath, 262
bean, 61, 186, 196–197
Belviq (lorcaserin HCL), 249
beta-blocker, 160t–161t
beta-cell, 10–11
beta-glucan, 323t
beverage, 18t, 144–145, 179
Bifidobacterium, 326
biguanide, 55t, 85, 109
bile acid sequestrant, 183t
biofeedback, 257
birthday, 238
bitter melon, 324t
bladder, 256, 294
bleeding, 274
blindness, 311–312
blood clot, 305t
blood glucose level. *See also* A1C;
    hyperglycemia; hypoglycemia
    alcohol, 76
    carbohydrate effect on, 34
    dental hygiene, 119
    diabetes diagnosis, 12–13
    dining out, 73
    exercise, 140–142
    fluctuations, 131–134
    food choices, 16
    fruit, 59
    high blood pressure, 158
    hospitalization, 291–293
    humor, 120
    illness, 90
    insulin-to-carbohydrate ratio, 219–224
    kidneys, 114–115
    metformin, 85
    sexual problems, 191
    skin care, 270
    Symlin (Pramlintide Acetate), 268
    target range, 25–26
    weight, 149, 153, 202
blood glucose monitor, 23–24
blood pressure, 82–84, 115–116, 158,
    231, 259–261

blood pressure monitor, 194–195
blood transfusion, 298
blood urea nitrogen (BUN), 115
blood vessel, 82
blurry vision, 311
Bodhi Day, 239
body hair, 274
body mass index (BMI), 151, 152t,
    179, 249
bolus insulin, 310
Boxing Day, 240
brain, 34
bread, 17t
breast, 294
breast cancer, 305t
breast-feeding, 269
brown adipose tissue, 149
bruising, 274
Buddha's Enlightenment, 239
Bureau of Primary Health Care, 67
butter, 101
Bydureon, 137t
Byetta, 137t

C

C reactive protein, 120
caffeine, 144, 320
calcium, 126–127, 199
calcium channel blockers (CCBs),
    160t–161t
calorie, 38–39, 99, 150, 177t–178t, 202
Calorie King, 234t
calorie-free, 42
Campbell, Colin, 302
cancer, 198, 294
cannabidiol (CBD), 264
carb impact, 128
carbohydrate, 16, 34–43, 76, 91, 110,
    126–130, 227–228, 308–309
cardiac stress test, 21, 231
cardiovascular disease (CVD), 82, 104,
    118, 183, 230–232, 302, 305t
cardiovascular risk, 39, 76, 120, 231, 303
cataract, 311
celebration, 238–240
celiac disease, 252–253
cell, 196